Praise for **Mindful Self-Compassion for Burnout**

"When we're pushed beyond our limits, self-compassion is the most overlooked—yet crucial—medicine we have for regaining resilience, wise perspective, and wholehearted engagement with life. Drawing on their experience as global leaders in the field of self-compassion, Drs. Neff and Germer have created an invaluable toolkit filled with powerful, actionable strategies to transform your relationship with stress."

—TARA BRACH, PHD, author of *Radical Acceptance*

"What a helpful book! It is almost like you are sitting with Drs. Neff and Germer and feeling their kindness and support. You learn about the science of burnout, and how to recover and even grow from it. With stories, practical exercises, deep insights, and lots of encouragement, you are guided step by step to real well-being and open-hearted ways to manage the challenges of life."

—RICK HANSON, PHD, author of *Resilient*

"This book has been a game-changer for me as far as understanding my burnout patterns and replacing self-criticism with compassionate self-talk. I feel less emotionally exhausted and more connected with myself and my patients."

—ALEXIS R., emergency room nurse, San Diego

"Drs. Neff and Germer offer practical strategies and profound insights that can help you cultivate resilience and reclaim your vitality. This book not only helps you recover from burnout, but also empowers you to thrive."

—JAMES R. DOTY, MD, Founder and Director,
Center for Compassion and Altruism Research
and Education, Stanford University School of Medicine

"A 'must read' for anyone seeking support and renewal, this book helps you navigate the high demands of our world with tender-hearted wisdom. Through scientific research, mindful self-compassion practices, and poignant personal examples, Drs. Neff and Germer illuminate a path for meeting burnout with kindness, mindfulness, and shared humanity."

—SHARON SALZBERG, author of *Lovingkindness* and *Real Life*

"This book arrived with perfect timing—I was emerging from a period of burnout and seeking more mindfulness in my life. It reads like a warm note from a good friend. This book definitely belongs in my daily toolkit for adapting and thriving as a highly sensitive person in today's world."

—CLIFF A., Cambridge, Massachusetts

"This book skillfully weaves together wisdom, scientific insights, and relatable stories. It helps you recognize and navigate burnout. By normalizing this common struggle, the authors provide a roadmap for healing and personal growth."

—RICHARD GOERLING, founder, Mindful Badge Initiative; retired police lieutenant and military veteran

MINDFUL SELF-COMPASSION FOR BURNOUT

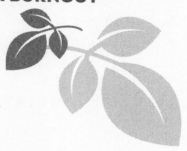

Also Available

MINDFUL SELF-COMPASSION FOR BURNOUT

Tools to Help You Heal
and Recharge When You're
Wrung Out by Stress

Kristin Neff, PhD
Christopher Germer, PhD

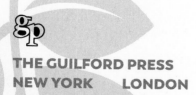

THE GUILFORD PRESS
NEW YORK   LONDON

Copyright © 2024 The Guilford Press
A Division of Guilford Publications, Inc.
370 Seventh Avenue, Suite 1200, New York, NY 10001
www.guilford.com

Printed in the United States of America

Last digit is print number: 9 8 7 6 5 4 3 2 1

Library of Congress Cataloging-in-Publication Data

Names: Neff, Kristin, author. | Germer, Christopher K., author.
Title: Mindful self-compassion for burnout : tools to help you heal
   and recharge when you're wrung out by stress / Kristin Neff, PhD,
   Christopher Germer, PhD.
Description: New York : The Guilford Press, [2024] | Includes
   bibliographical references and index.
Identifiers: LCCN 2024026572 | ISBN 9781462550227 (paperback) |
   ISBN 9781462554980 (hardcover)
Subjects: LCSH: Burn out (Psychology) | Stress (Psychology) | Self-
   acceptance. | Compassion. | Mindfulness (Psychology) | BISAC:
   SELF-HELP / Personal Growth / Happiness | SOCIAL SCIENCE /
   Social Work
Classification: LCC BF481 .N33 2024 | DDC 158.7/23—dc23/
   eng/20240703
LC record available at *https://lccn.loc.gov/2024026572*

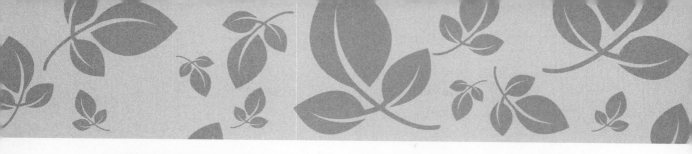

CONTENTS

ACKNOWLEDGMENTS

This is the third book we've written together, and the number of people who have contributed to the field of self-compassion research and practice, and the Mindful Self-Compassion (MSC) program in particular, has grown steadily throughout this time. We're so grateful for everyone's efforts, and especially grateful to those who are practicing self-compassion to transform their own lives and the lives of others. That's the foundation we're standing on today.

As anyone who has written a book knows, the energy behind a book is often a personal struggle that the author is trying to resolve. Therefore, when Kristin first proposed the idea of this book given our own struggles with burnout, we thought, "Great idea, but we're too burned out to do it on our own. Let's find a ghostwriter to help." Much to our amazement, our brilliant editor at The Guilford Press, Chris Benton, who shepherded *The Mindful Self-Compassion Workbook* to completion, was willing to try. We hammered out a detailed outline, and Chris B. wrote a rough first draft. This made it much easier for us to rewrite the book once we got our mojo back and saved us from staring at a blank page. We also kept much of Chris B.'s witty prose from her original effort. Afterward, Chris B. edited what we had written and tied the manuscript together and put a bow on it. There is no chance this book would have happened without Chris Benton. We're grateful not only for her writing and editing talent, but also for her encouragement, patience, and equanimity during the writing process. (Hopefully we didn't burn her out!) Deep bow to Chris B.

We would also like to thank Kitty Moore, our editor and publisher at Guilford, who has been championing self-compassion for years. Her excitement about this project sustained us from the beginning, and since she and Chris B. have been close friends and colleagues for almost two decades, we can only imagine the timely support and encouragement she gave to Chris at critical junctures. Our team had depth. Other valued members of the team at The Guilford Press were Anna Brackett, our supercareful Editorial Project Manager; Paul Gordon, Art Director, who makes all books a joy to behold; Bethanne Steneck, who made the pages look beautiful; Andrea Lansing, Lucy Baker, Katie Leonard, and others on the marketing team, who make sure our efforts are not for naught; and Rosalie Wieder, copyeditor.

We would like to acknowledge Krista Gregory, who awarded Kristin a grant to develop the Self-Compassion for Healthcare Communities (SCHC) program and was instrumental in discovering how self-compassion can prevent burnout in health care workers. We are also grateful to Drs. Phoebe Franco and Marissa Knox, who were part of the team that developed SCHC and still teach it to this day. In addition, we're grateful to our friends at the Center for Mindful Self-Compassion who are taking SCHC out into the larger world, especially Natalie Bell, Paula Gardiner, MD, and Elizabeth Lin, MD.

On a personal note, I (Kristin) would like to acknowledge the support of my family and friends, who provided such joy and meaning to my life as I was writing this book. I (Chris) am especially grateful for the support of my wife, Claire, who helped me navigate the crucible of burnout and then accompanied me over the bumps of the writing process.

Finally, we'd like to honor the courage of readers who have picked up this book. It takes guts to admit when we're burned out, and even more guts to turn *toward* burnout with curiosity and a commitment to do something about it. We don't take this for granted, and we wish you a safe and fruitful journey.

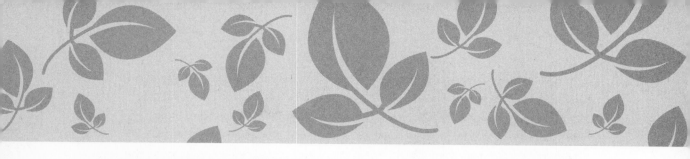

INTRODUCTION

What brought you to this book? If it was the word *burnout*, you're probably:

- Tired of feeling stressed out every day
- Tired of people expecting too much from you
- Tired of having too little impact, despite caring so much and working so hard
- Tired of trying to "do it all" and to "have it all"

Maybe you're Just. Plain. Tired.

The term *burnout* is so prevalent these days that its meaning has been somewhat diluted. People say things like "I'm burned out on Zoom calls" or "I'm burned out on politics." But for those who are truly experiencing *burnout,* it's not just a buzzword. It's a debilitating syndrome that makes it hard to get through each day because you're so drained, exhausted, and numb.

If the problem of burnout is all too familiar to you, you may be intrigued by our solution: *self-compassion.* This benevolent mindset can help you rekindle an active, vibrant life. Self-compassion involves relating to your emotional distress—including feeling like an epic failure—with warmth, understanding, and support. You might worry that self-compassion means blowing off responsibility for your mistakes, undermining your ability to correct them. But the opposite is true; self-compassion helps you take personal responsibility for your missteps and is a more effective motivator of change than harsh self-criticism.

Burnout gets worse when we suppress our pain and try to just stiff-upper-lip it. Self-compassion provides the sense of care and safety needed to feel the pain of burnout and move on from it. We also make burnout worse when we blame ourselves for our sorry state. Self-compassion tells us that the experience of burnout is natural and normal, that we're not alone, and that we are worthy of love and kindness as we heal and recover.

This is not a book about burnout per se. You already know you're burned out, and there are dozens of great books out there explaining what burnout is and what causes it. This is a toolkit that provides easy ways to practice self-compassion when you feel you can't carry on a moment longer. So what does self-compassion for burnout look like? Let's look first at what self-compassion for burnout is *not*.

It's not "self-care"—you know, that list of small acts you can do for yourself presented in employer-mandated webinars and on "wellness" websites. You don't need to be handed that list again. (Hot baths? *Please.* Sleep better? *When?* Eat right? *Who's doing the cooking—to say nothing of the grocery shopping?*) It's not advice to simply do less, as often offered by well-meaning family and friends. ("Can't you just let go of a few things?" *Like what—the kids, the house, the paycheck?*) It's not I'm-okay-you're-okay pablum. The point is when you're burned out, you're *not* okay, and being told you should feel okay implies you should just suck it up.

Self-compassion is a mindset shift that helps you relate to your burnout in a kinder, more productive way. It can be developed through a set of concrete, learnable skills that you practice in the middle of daily life and that don't require extra time out of your schedule.

The purpose of self-compassion is not to make you feel better. *Self-compassion changes the way you deal with the distress of burnout* so that you stop avoiding it, beating yourself up for it, or judging yourself as somehow deficient because you can't do it all. If you're a professional caregiver, it's a way to keep caring for your patients without sacrificing yourself. If you're an overworked family caregiver, it's a way to do your best for your family without letting resentment engulf your love. If you're the last to leave your workplace every day, it's a way to keep being productive without feeling like an empty water dispenser.

Ours is a demanding world. Self-compassion can help us stop harshly judging ourselves for the fact that we all struggle. But the power of self-compassion is not confined to our internal lives. When you cultivate the habit of self-compassion, you will find that it helps open your eyes to new ways to change and grow. Self-compassion involves both tender acceptance of ourselves and fierce action in the world. It helps us draw boundaries in the face of impossible demands and unrealistic expectations and spurs us to create a more just home life, workplace, and community.

Fortunately, this stuff works. In 2003 I (Kristin) created a scale to measure self-compassion called (unsurprisingly) the Self-Compassion Scale and published the first study examining the link between self-compassion and well-being. There are now thousands of studies confirming the benefits of self-compassion in general, as well as hundreds of studies establishing the benefits of self-compassion for alleviating burnout in particular. (We will be sprinkling these research findings throughout this book.)

In 2010 we jointly created the eight-session Mindful Self-Compassion program (MSC) to help people be more self-compassionate in their daily life. We later adapted the MSC practices to help health care professionals cope with burnout (see Chapter 2). Because they worked so effectively, we decided to create this toolkit of self-compassion practices to help people from all walks of life who were struggling with burnout. This includes us, since we've also teetered on the edge of burnout.

For me (Kristin), it was the stress of parenting a special-needs teen during the pandemic that tapped me out. My son's father moved to Germany after our divorce in 2018 and I had no family in town, so I was effectively on my own. Just as COVID hit, my son developed OCD (on top of autism and anxiety) and started having real mental health issues. You can imagine what it was like trying to find him the right treatment, oversee his schooling, and teach my university classes while everything was shut down. I relied on self-compassion to get me through, and I can't imagine how I would have coped without it. The ability to support myself with warmth and encouragement during the darkest of days meant that even though I was scared and exhausted like everyone else, I wasn't derailed by the stress. I was able to be there for my son without losing myself in the process, thanks to self-compassion.

For me (Chris), the struggle with burnout was partly a phase-of-life issue. I'm seventy-one years old now, and a couple years ago it became clear to me that I might have only ten or twenty years left to live. "What's it going to be?" I thought. I felt an intense urge to spend more time meditating and less time seeing patients, attending meetings, and teaching, but that wasn't happening. I had a book project that wasn't getting off the ground, and I felt irritated when people asked me to do work-related tasks for them. I'm an accommodating person by nature, but during this crunch time, tender self-compassion said to me, "Yes, you *must* follow your deepest desires," and fierce self-compassion told me, "You can do it. Your world will not collapse. Just don't schedule any work stuff before noon." Well, now two years later, after I meditate to my heart's content in the morning, I find that most things I do after noon are pretty enjoyable. I'm still working a lot, but in a different way, and my wife thinks I've become a happier person. In other words, I responded to early signs of burnout—procrastination, irritability, and malaise—with self-compassion, and it changed my life for the better.

We both realized how powerful self-compassion was for dealing with feelings of burnout, so we decided to write this book so that others could also benefit.

Each chapter in this book offers one self-compassion practice that we call a "tool." This terminology is intentional, as the practice is not one extra thing you need to *do* on top of your already insane to-do list. Instead, each tool is something you can *use* to lighten the emotional load of burnout when difficult moments arise throughout your day. Each chapter also tells the story of one person suffering burnout and how the tool helped the healing process begin. (These stories are composites; the individuals' personal details, including demographic information, have been altered to protect their identities.)

Ideally you should read the chapters in order because later skills build on earlier ones, but you can skip around if some chapters draw you in more than others. The book contains some theory and research, but it's mainly a guide to practicing self-compassion. You need to use the tools to see how they work. We won't tell you that self-compassion is magic dust that will make your burnout disappear, but we can promise that it will help you get through each day with greater strength and resilience.

So let's begin.

WHEN YOUR CUP RUNS DRY

The Causes and Consequences of Burnout

The word *burnout* calls up the image of a flame gasping for the last bit of available oxygen; dying embers or cold ashes; a spent fire that no longer keeps you warm and safe. It also vividly captures the experience of people like Jacquie.

Jacquie is slumped in the front seat of her car, parked in her driveway, after a grueling shift at the hospital. She feels like a melon scraped to the rind. She can't move—hell, she's not even sure she can breathe—and so she just sits there. She's been late for work five times in the last few months, more than in her prior twelve years as a critical care nurse. She used to love going to work and helping her patients recover and restart their lives, but now they seem like annoyances rather than people. She feels lame and useless and is having trouble doing basic tasks that used to be second nature to her, like putting in IVs. The only thing that gets her to the hospital each day is knowing that her coworkers, just as exhausted, would have to cover for her if she didn't show up.

If you were to tell Jacquie that she needs to give herself some compassion, she would probably throw her orthopedic shoe at you. "Don't you get it? I don't have an ounce of compassion left to give! My cup is completely dry!" She doesn't realize that compassion must flow inward as well as outward for it to be sustainable. This is nonnegotiable. When we care for others but ignore our own needs, feeling drained is inevitable. In fact, self-compassion is key to both preventing and recovering from burnout. In Latin, *passion* means "to suffer" and *com* means "with." We need to learn how to be with our own stress and exhaustion with kindness and support so that it doesn't overwhelm us.

This book will provide a variety of tools to help you do just that, drawn from the eight-week Mindful Self-Compassion (MSC) course. MSC is taught all over the world and contains many tools and techniques that have been scientifically proven to increase self-compassion and reduce burnout. The good news is these practices can be used at any moment in daily life and don't take a lot of time or effort.

Before delving further into what self-compassion is and how to develop it, we need to take a closer look at the causes and consequences of burnout. *Burnout* is a fitting (if graphic) metaphor when you look at how someone like Jacquie feels. If you picked up this book, the word is also likely to describe your experience. While not defined as a disease or a psychiatric disorder, burnout can be just as damaging as a disease. The exhaustion you feel can make it hard to get through the day. The loss of passion for your work can leave you numb and empty. And the inability to get things done the way you used to takes its toll on your self-image and personal fulfillment, to say nothing of the hit your productivity takes.

The phenomenon we now call *burnout* has been acknowledged by one name or another for centuries, but only in the last fifty years has it captured the attention of psychologists and public health organizations. "Burnout" was coined in 1974 by clinical psychologist Herbert Freudenberger, who noticed the toll that working in a free clinic for drug addicts had on him and other volunteers. According to surveys, between one-third and three-quarters of people worldwide are burned out in their current work, whether it's paid employment or unpaid labor such as caring for children or elderly parents. (Throughout this book, we'll be using the term *work* to refer to both.) That's an astounding number. Whether burnout is actually more common than it once was or we're just more aware of it is difficult to assess accurately, but there's no doubt that it infects all sectors of

Burnout is typically defined by these three symptoms:

Exhaustion—feeling drained and fatigued with nothing left to give

Depersonalization—feeling detached, cynical, or negative about your work

Reduced accomplishment—feeling ineffective, inept, or incompetent

society. We can see it in any situation where stress is high and people are working really hard to reach goals that they care deeply about:

- Health care professionals (who are tasked with saving lives yet can spend more time shuffling papers than taking care of patients)
- Teachers (who must meet the vocal and conflicting demands of parents, students, administrators, and school boards)
- Employees in fast-paced businesses (who are expected to be on call 24/7 and never get a break from their phones or computer screens)
- Members of the clergy (who may have bottomless devotion to their flock but bottomed-out resources for counseling them)
- Police and other emergency responders (who must make life-and-death decisions in five-alarm fires, drug overdoses, and mass shootings)
- Civil servants (who signed up to serve their country, state, city, or town but are receiving death threats from conspiracy-fueled crazies)
- Therapists and social workers (who are faced with the worst of human struggles and listen to devastating life stories day after day)
- Social justice or climate activists (who fight for the greater good yet find progress achingly slow)
- Adults caring for ailing parents (who may have to support, feed, dress, and bathe their own parents in a complete role reversal)
- Parents raising high-needs children (who provide heroic care but are overwhelmed and worried about their kids' future)

ARE YOU BURNED OUT?

To determine whether you're currently experiencing burnout, ask yourself the following questions:

- ☐ Are you less motivated to do your work?
- ☐ Are you always stressed and feel you never get a break?

- ❑ Do you find yourself becoming impatient or irritable?
- ❑ Are you less productive, or does it feel that way?
- ❑ Do you have difficulty concentrating?
- ❑ Do you feel hopeless or overwhelmed?
- ❑ Is work stress spilling into your personal relationships?
- ❑ Do you just want to be left alone?
- ❑ Are you starting to use food, alcohol, or drugs to numb the stress you feel?
- ❑ Is your work affecting your sleep or your sex life?
- ❑ Are you becoming anxious or depressed about your work?
- ❑ Are you developing physical problems, like headaches or stomach problems?

If you answered yes to four or five of these questions, it's no wonder you're looking for help. Burnout typically starts with exhaustion from a specific stressor (in an occupational space or at home) but then seeps into the rest of your life.

Burnout can cause physical problems such as fatigue, body aches, headaches, heart disease, appetite changes, diabetes, stomach or bowel problems, and vulnerability to illnesses. Especially when unaddressed, burnout can have a profound impact on mental health, leading to anxiety, depression, or substance abuse. We are also not our best selves with other people, perhaps getting angry over nothing or isolating ourselves from friends and family. Any of these symptoms of burnout can have a devastating effect on our lives.

> **To learn more about the signs and symptoms of burnout**, you can consult the American Psychological Association website (*apa.org*), the World Health Organization (*who.int*), or WebMD (*webmd.com*).

Burnout can affect all aspects of your life, leaving you feeling as flat as a deflated balloon.

It's also no surprise that burnout can have an insidious effect on society at large. Nurses and teachers are starting to check out, often leaving the profession. The last few years have seen record numbers of Americans quit their jobs—several million a month. Analysts report that many are exiting due to burnout, especially health care workers. This only increases the burden on those who stay, who feel more burned out than ever.

Employee turnover costs billions of dollars to institutions in Europe and the United States—employers estimate that about one-third of an employee's annual salary per year is lost to burnout. Some companies can't afford this cost and close shop. Others pass on the cost to consumers, who can't afford it either. And what happens to all of us when there's a long wait for a 911 response; your priest, imam, or rabbi needs *your* counsel; and marginalized individuals can't get the social services they need to survive? You know the answer because all of us are living with the far-reaching consequences of burnout.

You might also be asking yourself the question "How did I get so burned out in the first place?" This is a good question to ask if you're trying to decide whether you can continue in the work you're doing—work that was probably very meaningful to you at one time.

THE CAUSES OF BURNOUT

You might not even be able to remember how the great drain began. Burnout can lead to cognitive and memory problems to the point that things become a blur. When asked if he remembered a big snowstorm in 2021, one high school teacher, exhausted by having to switch suddenly to teaching online due to the COVID pandemic, replied: "To be honest, I don't remember a thing about last year." But scientists have linked burnout with several identifiable factors.

Work-Related Stressors

- **Excessive workload:** You have too much to do, can never catch up, your work is physically or emotionally exhausting.

- **Lack of control:** You are unable to make your own decisions, control your schedule, or solve problems your own way.

- **Unclear work expectations:** You're confused about what's expected and who does what.

- **Limited rewards:** You're poorly paid or inadequately recognized for your work.

- **Unfairness:** Your personal identity or intersections of identity are marginalized or disrespected, or policies and procedures are administered inequitably.

- **Dysfunctional workplace:** You experience bullying, micromanaging, undermining.

- **Lack of support:** You feel isolated, lack community, or experience job insecurity.

- **Distressing work:** Your work is monotonous, chaotic, dangerous, or demeaning.

- **Values conflict:** Your work violates your core values (also known as *moral injury*).

Any one of these conditions can lead to burnout, but burnout usually results from a combination of factors. For example, being a critical care nurse is hard enough, but Jacquie, unfortunately, also feels completely disrespected by a profit-driven hospital administration that refuses to hire the additional staff it needs. She spends so much time doing paperwork that she can spend only a few minutes with each patient personally. She hasn't received a decent raise in years, yet her rent keeps going up. All these stressors pile up like a multicar crash.

Caring

Research shows that deeply caring about one's job is also a risk factor for burnout. An idealistic person who starts a homeless shelter and who is passionate about aiding those at the margins of society will work tirelessly for clients. But they may also become bitter and disillusioned about the dehumanizing attitude of those holding both the purse strings and the pens that write public policy. If they didn't care, the frustrations of the job wouldn't weigh on them so heavily. Ironically, it's those who are most committed to their work who are most vulnerable to being drained by it.

Imbalance

Work–life imbalance is also a key risk factor for burnout, and many of us fall victim to it. We receive cultural messages that we're supposed to work hard and *love* what we do: "If you love the work you do, you never have to work a day in your life!" Somehow this gets subconsciously translated into "If you love the work you do, never live a day without work!" As people increasingly find themselves working online and from home, it's becoming more and more difficult to step away from work and focus on other things. The boss is only an email message away, so work starts taking time away from friends or family, warping its role in our lives even further.

This tug-of-war between work and family is especially strong for women. Sure, second-wave feminism bestowed on women the "right" to "have it all," but here we are in the fourth wave and women still feel guilty about not spending enough time caring for their families. Before Ketanji Brown Jackson took her seat on the U.S. Supreme Court, she felt the need to acknowledge to her daughters that she hadn't always gotten the work–mom balance right. There she was, being confirmed as the first Black woman on the highest court in the United States, and she was still worried that she hadn't done enough.

In dual-earner households, women tend to do twice as much child care and housework as men. They also spend more time coordinating family activities, planning celebrations, arranging doctor visits, checking in on relatives, and so on. The result is that four in ten working mothers report always feeling rushed, with little to no time left for themselves. And those who earn more than their male partners actually increase rather than decrease their unpaid labor to make up for the perception that they somehow aren't being good women. This self-judgment just makes feelings of burnout worse.

Self-Worth

Our sense of self-worth often comes from how productive we are: "I'm most valuable when I'm working hard." This is true for most people, but especially for perfectionists, for whom good enough is never good enough. Our society tells us we should always be trying to achieve more. Instead of stopping work when a task is completed, we keep going, trying to be better and better. Unfortunately, achievement only makes us feel better for a few moments, and then it's back to the treadmill. This sense of never being productive enough eventually causes us to feel empty and depleted.

Self-Sacrifice

People tend to burn out when they focus on caring for others much more than themselves. Self-sacrifice is seen as admirable and noble. Those raised as women, especially, are praised for being self-sacrificing to the point where it becomes part of their identity. The whole reason Jacquie went into nursing was to help people. But she became so identified with the idea of being a "helpful person" that she was afraid to say no to her colleagues, working extra shifts even when she was so tired that she could barely stand. When we care for others but not ourselves, burnout is sure to follow.

Self-Blame

Feelings of stress and exhaustion are multiplied exponentially when we judge and blame ourselves for our predicament. Our inner critic says we should be able to control things, to get it right, to handle it. When we lose steam and start disconnecting from our work, self-blame just makes us feel inept and incapable. Not only am I failing at my job, I *am* a failure, a loser, a lost cause. We point the finger at ourselves in the misplaced hope that somehow it will give us the kick in the butt needed to pull ourselves out of burnout. But it just digs the trench deeper.

If you're burned out, you don't need self-blame. You need self-compassion.

If you tell yourself that you wouldn't feel this way if you were a better person—tougher, thicker-skinned, more dedicated, more generous, a harder worker—you're mistaken. Your working conditions are beating you up every day, and it won't help matters to pummel yourself further. It's time to try something new. What would it be like to validate how painful it is to feel burned out; to remind yourself that you're a human being doing the best you can and you're not alone; to be kind to yourself because burnout hurts and you're suffering? In other words, how might self-compassion help you cope with burnout?

Self-Compassion Assessment

To decide for yourself whether self-compassion might help you with burnout, please take this test, which is based on the empirically validated Self-Compassion Scale.

How Do I Relate to Being Burned Out?

Read each statement carefully before answering. To the left of each item, indicate how often you behave in the stated manner when you feel stressed, exhausted, and burned out.

For the first set of items, use the following scale:

Almost never	Occasionally	Sometimes	Frequently	Almost always
1	2	3	4	5

____ I try to be understanding and patient toward myself.

____ I try to take a balanced view of the situation.

____ I try to see my experience as part of the human condition.

____ I try to give myself the caring and tenderness I need.

____ I try to keep my emotions in balance.

____ I try to remind myself that difficult feelings are shared by most people.

For the next items, use the following scale (which differs from the one above):

Almost always	Frequently	Sometimes	Occasionally	Almost never
1	2	3	4	5

____ I'm disapproving and judgmental about myself.

____ I become consumed by negative feelings.

____ I tend to feel like most other people are probably happier than I am.

____ I'm intolerant and impatient toward myself.

____ I tend to feel all alone.

____ I tend to obsess and fixate on everything that's wrong.

Total (sum of all 12 items) _____

Mean score = Total/12 _____

Average overall self-compassion scores tend to be around 3.0 on the 1–5 scale, so you can interpret your overall score accordingly. As a rough guide, a score of 1–2.5 for your overall self-compassion indicates you are low in self-compassion for burnout, 2.5–3.5 indicates you are moderate, and 3.5–5.0 means you are high in self-compassion.

Jacquie took the assessment and realized she gave herself very little compassion for feeling burned out. Since she was a research-oriented type, she went ahead and read the studies showing that self-compassion reduces feelings of exhaustion, detachment, and incompetence and decided she wanted to give it a try.

This book provides concrete tools for folks like Jacquie, and perhaps you, to relate to burnout in a healthier and more productive way. As you'll learn in the next chapter, self-compassion can significantly ease the mental, physical, and emotional impact of burnout. Self-compassion can also help restore your passion for your work, allowing you to continue fighting the good fight.

No matter how long you may have suffered from burnout or how hopeless you may feel, self-compassion can meet you right where you are. Anyone can practice self-compassion, and it won't take any more of your limited time and energy. In fact, a moment of real self-compassion is always a relief—a mini-vacation from the struggle of burnout. The next chapter will help you understand what self-compassion is and how it can help you. Why not try it out and see what happens?

2

REPLENISHING OURSELVES

How Self-Compassion Combats Burnout

Self-compassion is pretty straightforward—it's simply compassion turned inward. When we're self-compassionate, we give ourselves the same kindness, care, concern, and help when we struggle that we typically give to others. We're warm and understanding rather than cold and judgmental when things are challenging in our lives.

Scientists define compassion as concern with the alleviation of suffering. It's the motivation to help rather than harm. We tend to do this quite naturally for *other* people we care about; less so for ourselves. Take Laurel, for instance.

Laurel works from home as a computer programmer, but she recently acquired another job—caring for her mother, who is eighty-seven. After Laurel's father passed away, her mom felt derailed by the loss, so she moved into the spare room in Laurel's house. Her mom has trouble walking and is losing her sight and hearing, so Laurel helps her bathe, drives her to doctors' appointments, and cooks for her. Laurel is overwhelmed by how much time she's spending caring for her mom while trying to work full-time. She's the only child, so has no help from siblings. When she suggested to her mom that she move into assisted living, Mom was clearly hurt. Although her mom said she'd be willing, she obviously hated the idea. Laurel immediately took back the suggestion: "Never mind, I'm happy to take care of you, Mom." Laurel feels like a bad daughter for wanting her mom to move out. She also feels incompetent. Shouldn't she be better able to juggle working from home with caregiving? To deal with her shame and feelings of inadequacy, she's started drinking a bit too much in the evenings after her mom goes to bed.

When we're burned out—exhausted, depleted, fed up—the last thing we need is shame and blame. Shame just makes us feel more exhausted, depleted, and fed up. We need a helping hand rather than a slap across the face. Compassion helps us get through a difficult situation by offering support and encouragement, which energizes rather than drains us.

Luckily, by the time we've reached adulthood, most of us already know how to be compassionate, at least toward others. We know how to be there for someone who needs us—to listen empathically, to talk things through, and to help out when we can. For instance, even though Laurel doesn't feel up to the task of caring for her mom, she's one of the most patient, caring, and protective daughters you'd ever want. She sticks up for her mom when others talk down to her: when her doctor recently spoke to her mother in a condescending way, Laurel blurted, "She's hard of hearing, not ignorant!" Laurel also tells her mom how much she loves her and holds Mom's hand when she feels scared or lonely. If Laurel gave herself half the kindness and understanding that she gives to her mom, she would probably feel very differently about herself.

Self-compassion can answer the needs of burned-out people like Laurel (shown in the box on the facing page). Is its impact exaggerated? Not at all. As described later in this chapter, scientists have a ton of evidence that self-compassion can help reduce burnout. If you're running on empty, it may be a relief to know that you don't need to learn a brand-new skill to be self-compassionate. You just need to reach into your back pocket and take out the tool you already know how to use with others—compassion—and begin to treat yourself like you would a good friend.

RESISTANCE TO SELF-COMPASSION

A major block to being self-compassionate, however, is that we don't give ourselves permission to be kind to ourselves. "Compassion for *myself*?" protested Laurel, "How can I feel sorry for myself when my mother is nearing the end of her life? My duty as her daughter is to take care of her, not to wallow in self-pity because it's hard work."

This type of self-talk comes from many different messages we've heard over our lives. We're told we should be tough and interpret that to mean we should be harsh and callous toward ourselves. If you were raised in a negligent or abusive

Giving Ourselves What We Need

When you're burned out, you can ask yourself the quintessential self-compassion question, "What do I need right now?" Then do what you can to meet your needs. Maybe you resonate with one of these needs commonly experienced by people who are burned out:

✦ **Acceptance**: "So you're not perfect at your job. That's okay. Who's perfect anyway?"

✦ **Comfort**: How would you soothe and comfort a friend who is feeling exhausted and overwhelmed? You can offer the same care to yourself.

✦ **Validation**: It's healing to admit that burnout feels really bad and you need some support.

✦ **Boundaries**: Learning to say no can help you lighten the load so that you aren't taking on more than you can handle.

✦ **Speaking up**: Part of self-compassion is standing up for yourself and expressing how you really feel.

✦ **Fulfillment**: Ask yourself what would help you feel replenished, and then do what you can to make that happen.

✦ **Change**: Become a wise, encouraging coach toward yourself as you attempt to make changes in your life so you're less overwhelmed.

atmosphere, or you grew up without the inner security and validation that comes from consistent, responsive care from a parent, you might carry a sense of worthlessness into your adult life. You may secretly feel that you don't deserve compassion. The fact that you're exhausted and burned out seems only to prove the point—you don't measure up, and therefore your needs don't matter. This is Laurel's story. When she's worn out after a long day of work and wants to put off giving her mom a bath until the morning, she hears the critical voice of her father in her head, telling her how lazy she is.

Society's messages echo loudly as well. Part of Laurel's resistance to self-compassion is rooted in the culture in which she (along with many others) was raised, which lauded self-sacrifice as noble and even saintly—especially for women. She built her sense of self around being generous and giving. And now, unfortunately, with the high demands of caring for her mom, her own needs keep sinking to the bottom. Laurel needs self-compassion to correct the imbalance in her habit of lopsided care, which always favors others over herself.

Burnout often results from lopsided care—favoring others over ourselves.

People have a lot of reasons for resisting self-compassion—they think it will make them weak, selfish, lazy, self-centered or self-indulgent, or that they'll avoid taking responsibility and won't get anything done. You'll have a chance to explore your misgivings about self-compassion more thoroughly in Chapter 4. But for now, we'd like to give you a better understanding of the rewards of using self-compassion to address burnout if you give it a try.

HOW SELF-COMPASSION HELPS: WHAT THE SCIENCE TELLS US

There is a lot of research on self-compassion and burnout, which has been conducted with health care professionals, emergency responders, teachers, therapists, educators, business leaders, employees, caregivers of elderly parents or spouses, and parents. Findings indicate that people who are naturally more self-compassionate, or who learn to be more self-compassionate, feel:

- Less exhausted and depleted by their work
- Less stressed and overwhelmed
- Less depressed, hopeless, or cynical
- More able to maintain a work–life balance
- Better able to draw boundaries with others
- More connected to others
- More able to cope with work challenges
- More competent and effective
- More satisfied with the work they do

Self-compassion can help protect you against the ravages of burnout.

Studies have also shown that people who are more self-compassionate benefit in terms of their general mental and physical health (see the box below). Studies are typically conducted by assessing natural levels of self-compassion using self-report measures like the Self-Compassion Scale and correlating scores with other outcomes, or else by examining what happens to those who learn to be more self-compassionate by taking a training course like MSC. Findings using both methods converge to demonstrate that self-compassion is very good for you.

The Benefits of Self-Compassion

People who are self-compassionate are more likely to:

✦ Be happy, hopeful, and optimistic
✦ Feel satisfied with their lives
✦ Have a stable and unconditional sense of self-worth
✦ Be appreciative of and satisfied with their bodies
✦ Have emotional intelligence
✦ Skillfully regulate their emotions
✦ Demonstrate resilience when faced with hardship
✦ Be conscientious and willing to take personal responsibility
✦ Show motivation and determination to reach their goals
✦ Focus on learning and personal growth
✦ Feel authentic in their social interactions
✦ Have healthy relationships with others
✦ Be forgiving and engage in perspective taking
✦ Eat healthy food, exercise, and get regular medical checkups
✦ Sleep well, have a strong immune system, and get fewer colds, aches, and pains

Self-compassionate people are also less likely to:

✦ Be neurotic or feel intense shame
✦ Be anxious, depressed, and stressed
✦ Abuse drugs and alcohol
✦ Engage in disordered eating
✦ Develop posttraumatic stress disorder
✦ Consider suicide as a way to escape emotional pain

CREATING A CULTURE OF SELF-COMPASSION

Several years ago (pre-COVID) a woman named Krista Gregory, who worked as a chaplain at a large children's hospital, took the MSC course that we developed. The course is taught in three-hour sessions that are held once a week for eight weeks. The training involves a variety of exercises that are practiced during class and between sessions as homework. It also includes a half-day silent meditation retreat. Krista was transformed by the experience and approached us to see if we could also help the overworked, stressed-out health care professionals at her hospital learn to be more self-compassionate. Her staff needed self-compassion desperately, but they didn't have time to take the full MSC course. "And don't even think about asking my staff to meditate or do self-compassion homework," Krista noted. "They barely have time to eat." So we started a pilot program, testing a self-compassion training for burned-out health care professionals.

There was some blowback at first. These folks were dealing with kids who had serious illnesses like cancer or juvenile diabetes. The culture of the hospital was all about sacrificing for the children. Nurses would work multiple shifts without a break. "Isn't self-compassion selfish?" they asked us. "Shouldn't we just be focusing on the kids?" Doctors felt the pressure to be perfect and never make a mistake because of the consequences if they did. Talk about stress. "Won't self-compassion make us sloppy and lazy and undermine how professional we are?" But everyone at the hospital trusted and respected Krista, and she talked some of her colleagues into helping us create the course.

We had to go through a few iterations until we found a format that worked. We created a version of the course that was much shorter—six one-hour sessions—and we taught it over lunch with free pizza (they had to eat, so might as well learn self-compassion while doing so). We also made sure that all the self-compassion practices could be done on the job, right on the spot at work, where they're needed. Many of the practices and techniques found in the book come directly from this course.

We conducted research on the efficacy of the brief training and found that the course not only raised self-compassion levels, it increased compassion for others. Our participants also reported more compassion satisfaction, meaning they felt more fulfilled by their work as health care professionals. They became more mindful on the job. They experienced a reduction in their stress and became less depressed. Perhaps most importantly, they reported significant reductions in the three core symptoms of burnout—they felt less exhausted and drained by their work; reported less detachment, cynicism, and negativity; and regained feelings of competence and effectiveness.

We had to think of a name for the program and decided to call it Self-Compassion for Healthcare Communities (SCHC). That was chosen because the program worked not only on the individual level but also at the community level and started to change the culture of the hospital. Those who took the course loved it and started to talk about their experience with others. They began to model a new way of approaching the stress of their jobs. Instead of just sucking it up, they would say, "I need to take a short break to care for myself right now." Even among those who hadn't taken the course, the idea that compassion should be given only to others started to shift. People began encouraging each other to be kinder and more understanding to themselves. They realized that they were no good to anyone if they were so exhausted that they couldn't think straight. They stopped expecting that everyone should be superhuman and instead began to embrace the fact that everyone was doing the best they could.

SCHC is still being taught at the children's hospital where it was developed, and it's also taught online through the Center for Mindful Self-Compassion, the nonprofit we started to disseminate self-compassion training. Many big health care organizations like Kaiser Permanente are starting to offer the program to their staff. Medical schools and residency programs are interested. People are finally starting to catch on to the fact that if you continually give to others and ignore yourself, you'll soon have nothing left to give. Most of us have learned over the years how to give compassion to friends, family, or colleagues when they're down. The good news is that you can draw on this experience to support yourself in a similar manner. We start the SCHC program with an exercise designed to provide insight into how we treat our friends and work colleagues, compared to ourselves, when we struggle. It's helpful to identify these differences, especially in the context of burnout, so that we can start being a better support to ourselves.

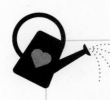

SELF-COMPASSION TOOL 2
How Would You Treat a Friend or Colleague Who Was Feeling Burned Out?

Please take out a sheet of paper (or your digital device) and reflect for a moment on the following questions:

✦ Imagine a close friend or colleague who revealed to you how exhausted and burned out they were feeling in their job, at home, or by life in general (this may have actually happened, of course). Also imagine that you were in a strong and centered space. *What would you say to this person? What tone would you use? What would your posture be like? Would you make any nonverbal gestures like putting a hand on a shoulder?*

✦ Now think about how you have responded to your own exhaustion and feelings of burnout. *What do you typically say to yourself? What tone do you use? What is your posture? Do you make any nonverbal gestures, like grimacing or clenching your fists?*

✦ Do you notice any differences between how you would treat a close friend or colleague and how you are treating yourself? Would you be kinder to someone else? Would you tell a friend it's not the end of the world to feel exhausted even though you catastrophize with yourself? Would you focus on situational factors with a colleague (the paperwork, other responsibilities) but just blame yourself for being burned out?

✦ Finally, see if you can respond to your feelings of burnout like you naturally would to someone you cared about. Try writing some words of kindness, understanding, and support in response to your situation, using the same warm, caring tone that you would use with a close friend or colleague.

Laurel didn't realize how badly she treated herself compared to how she would treat a friend who was overwhelmed. Laurel's friend Sarah worked full-time and had a son with autism, and Laurel was very kind and encouraging toward her. She constantly praised Sarah for being a loving mother and reminded her to cut herself some slack for not being able to do it all. She would never say to her friend, "You're not doing enough" or "It's your fault your son isn't doing better." Instead, she said things like "I'm so proud of you," "You're doing the best you can," and "It must be so hard. Is there anything I can do to help?"

When Laurel tried to say similar things to herself, it just felt uncomfortable and phony. You may have had a similar experience. That's very normal. In this book we'll help you work on being more compassionate toward yourself, and it will get easier with practice. Laurel continued trying to be friendlier to herself, and eventually it started to feel more natural. She was surprised at how much lighter she felt when she was able to let some of her own kindness in. She tried saying understanding things to herself like "I know it's really difficult to see Mom's decline and to feel so responsible for her, but you can't do it all. You're doing the best you can." Laurel realized that even though her mother might not be as happy in assisted living, it would probably be a better solution for both of them. It was just too stressful for Laurel to try to work from home and care for her mother at the same time. She wasn't a bad daughter for making this decision, even if her mom was hurt by it. Giving herself warmth and support in this way helped her get through this difficult time.

Luckily, self-compassion isn't rocket science. It primarily requires giving ourselves permission to invert the Golden Rule and "do unto ourselves as we would do unto others." Being hard on yourself, shaming yourself, and ignoring your needs makes it impossible to cope with the high-stakes demands of modern life. Learning to approach your stress in a friendlier and more supportive manner will give you the strength and resilience needed to recover from burnout. The next chapter dives into the elements of self-compassion so you can understand it in greater depth. You have the power to give yourself what you need to feel reenergized and whole again, if you're willing to give it a try.

3

A RECIPE FOR RESILIENCE

The Ingredients of Self-Compassion

There's no getting around it: burnout sucks. And yet "getting around it" is exactly what we try to do. We ignore our exhaustion, pretend we're not in pain, and batter ourselves with criticism to try to push forward. All of this is understandable: Who would want to feel burned out? But if we dropped these diversionary tactics for a second and asked ourselves, "How's that working for you?" the answer would be obvious. We're still stuck in burnout. And it still sucks.

When we're assaulted by stress at work or feel depleted, we need to tend to our distress. But caring for ourselves is rarely our immediate response. Instead of turning toward the pain, we muffle it. Instead of remembering how normal our feelings are, we feel all alone. Instead of being warm and supportive to ourselves, we're cold or even mean-spirited. We do all this because we don't want to feel bad, but ironically it just makes us feel worse.

Isaiah is the talented lifeblood of the software start-up he manages. Raised in a close-knit family that placed a huge value on working hard to get ahead, he often works seventy- to eighty-hour weeks and rarely takes a vacation. He used to have huge ambitions and wanted to be the next Microsoft. In the past he somehow kept his team going when they were in danger of falling short of their sales targets, as if he could move them forward through sheer willpower. But now he's tired of fighting—fighting for the investment funds to keep the business going, fighting to develop the next big thing before anyone else, fighting to make payroll for the twenty employees who depend on him to pay their rent. And he's becoming cranky as well as tired. Yesterday he snapped at his trustworthy assistant when she asked about a funding proposal that was due rather than flashing his usual dazzling smile. His assistant was so shocked that she burst into tears. Isaiah felt like a lowly reptile, not fit to call himself a leader. He's even started to withdraw from his husband, Jake, the person he has always counted on for support. He feels as if he's constantly pushing a boulder up a hill and is thinking of giving up and selling the company at a loss.

Self-compassion helps us care for ourselves when we're feeling burned out by providing the resources needed to turn *toward* our stress without being overwhelmed by it.

THE THREE COMPONENTS OF SELF-COMPASSION

There are three core components of self-compassion that work together to help us when we're struggling: mindfulness, common humanity, and self-kindness. Mindfulness allows us to be aware of our negative experiences with balance, clarity, and acceptance. Common humanity recognizes that everyone is imperfect and leads an imperfect life and that we aren't alone in our distress. Kindness involves giving ourselves the support and encouragement we need to help alleviate our suffering. These three elements are all necessary for resilience and coping. While they work together as a whole, each plays a specific role in the context of burnout.

> The three central elements of self-compassion are mindfulness, common humanity, and self-kindness.

Mindfulness: Being Aware of What Is

Mindfulness can be described as being aware of what's happening while it's happening. Think about how often your day goes by on autopilot. Especially if you're feeling burned out, you may feel like a zombie going from task to task, numb and cloudy inside. If you aren't aware of what you're feeling, how are you going to help yourself? Imagine if a friend called you up hoping for some comfort after a stressful workday. Your friend wants to tell you about what a difficult time they're having and how overwhelmed they are, but you don't listen to a word they say. That's how we often relate to our own stress: we simply ignore it. Many of us have been taught that ignoring or avoiding our difficult emotions is the better part of valor. "Giving in" to feelings of exhaustion or frustration will only stand in the way of getting things done, we believe. And we're reminded that there are plenty of people in the world who have it worse, so we shouldn't "wallow" in our suffering.

But ignoring how we're feeling means we can't answer the crucial question "What do I need in this moment to care for myself?" Do I need to take a break, draw a boundary, talk with colleagues, make a change, ask for a hug? Opening to the reality of the moment means we acknowledge that we're struggling and can say to ourselves, "This is really tough. I could use a little help right now."

As you'll discover in later chapters, mindfulness not only allows us to become aware of the pain of burnout, it also helps us lessen the resistance to it that is itself draining. When we accept our difficult feelings, the intensity of the pain actually decreases and we gain the perspective needed to respond wisely to our circumstances.

Common Humanity: Remembering That You're Not Alone

Burnout is one of the loneliest states we can end up in. Stress can shrink our world to a pinpoint as we focus on the work we need to get done. We don't have energy to spend time with others, so we may start to socially isolate ourselves. Or else we emotionally distance ourselves from those we're around because we feel so drained. The people we used to care about now seem like a burden, and we carry this burden alone.

Although logically we know that other people feel as we do, irrationally it can seem as if we're the only ones feeling so burned out. We feel as if everyone else in the world is leading a *normal* energetic, vibrant life. "Something must be wrong with me," we think. These thoughts are often hidden just below the surface of our awareness, where they remain unchallenged. And so our sense of being isolated in our own world persists.

This is what happened to Isaiah. He assumed that all his competitors were doing just fine emotionally and weren't as tired as he was. He was ashamed to admit how overwhelmed he was, so he tried to hide his distress from his employees and even Jake. He imagined that he was uniquely flawed and incompetent because he couldn't keep pulling the long hours, and this just made his feelings of isolation a hundred times worse.

When we're exhausted, detached, and battered by self-recrimination, remembering our shared humanity is more important than ever. First of all, the facts clearly show we aren't alone. Burnout is ubiquitous in society. It's only human that when stressed and overwhelmed long enough, we will begin to shut down in response. We aren't robots; we need rest and time to recuperate after a hard day. Feeling burned out doesn't mean there is something wrong with you. You're simply a human being doing the best you can in trying circumstances. A nurse who took our SCHC course reported being deeply moved by the concept of common humanity: "I used to build up so much tension telling myself that no one understood how hard my job was. And then there I was, looking around at a group of fifteen other staff who understood that perfectly, because they felt the same way. I felt myself exhale more deeply than I have in months."

Self-Kindness: Supporting and Caring for Yourself

When you're so burned out that you can't do your work anymore, it feels like you definitely don't have time to care for yourself. You might imagine that self-care means taking hour-long bubble baths or a yoga class. Self-kindness doesn't take time or effort—it just requires that you change your attitude toward yourself. Instead of judging and criticizing yourself for the dismal condition you're in, you try to be supportive and understanding, like you would be to a friend. Rather than giving yourself the cold shoulder because you feel somehow at fault for burning out, you're warm and benevolent. Think of yourself as a solar-powered battery. The sunlight of your care and concern recharges you, while the dark clouds of self-judgment and shame drain you.

Kindness isn't just a feeling, however; it's the active desire to alleviate your suffering. When you allow yourself to be moved by your feelings of exhaustion and burnout, your heart cracks open and the natural desire to help emerges. You begin to value your own well-being and want to *do something* about your situation. Like picking up this book—an act of self-kindness that will pay off sooner than you might think.

THE TWO FACES OF SELF-COMPASSION: TENDER AND FIERCE

Research shows that self-compassion helps us cope with difficult circumstances by embracing ourselves and our painful feelings, but also by changing the circumstances causing them. Tender self-compassion alleviates suffering through the power of acceptance. It has a gentle, nurturing quality that soothes and reassures us when we're distressed. But sometimes to care for ourselves we need to do something to end our distress—protect ourselves, fulfill our needs, or motivate change. This is where fierce self-compassion comes in. We alleviate suffering by taking action. Metaphorically speaking, tender self-compassion is like a mother holding and comforting her child while fierce self-compassion is like Mama Bear defending her cub. Fierce self-compassion involves setting boundaries, saying no, getting angry if needed to stand up for ourselves. It means we assert the right to get our needs met so that we don't give ourselves away. It also requires encouraging ourselves to learn and grow as individuals, while working to change unjust or harmful circumstances.

In the face of burnout, we need both tender and fierce self-compassion. We need to accept ourselves as an exhausted mess with great warmth and care so that we can begin to heal. We also need to call on our inner strength to protect ourselves from the forces draining us and to spur us forward so we can get back on our feet again. Like yin and yang, these two expressions of self-compassion must be balanced and integrated. If we're too accepting, we might become complacent and give up. But if we're too focused on taking action, we'll just wear ourselves out even more. We need to accept ourselves and our emotions while simultaneously working to change unhealthy behaviors and situations to recover fully from burnout.

Unfortunately, gender role socialization stands in the way of our ability to balance fierce and tender self-compassion. To be clear, the problem is not with what anatomy you were born with or your gender identity (whether you're a man, woman, or nonbinary). The problem is the shoebox that society places us in—how "men" and "women" are supposed to behave.

Women are encouraged to be tender and caring toward others but not themselves. They are rewarded for self-sacrifice and meeting others' needs while being eyed with suspicion when meeting their own needs. Women are also told they can't be too fierce—in other words strong, forceful, assertive, or powerful. Society doesn't like bossy, angry, or "ambitious" women. Gender role socialization means that women sometimes burn out because they don't feel comfortable drawing boundaries or saying no to others.

On the other hand, men are encouraged to be powerful and fierce but not sensitive or tender. In fact, young boys are often teased or bullied if they're too "sensitive," and this continues into adulthood. As a consequence, men may have less access to the healing power of self-compassion that comes from accepting or soothing their difficult emotions. They sometimes burn out because they fear easing up means being weak. Instead, they believe they should keep going like Rambo to prove their worth, ignoring the distress calls their bodies are making by shutting down with fatigue.

This was certainly the case with Isaiah. His approach to business was to keep working and never let up. He couldn't imagine taking a break or asking for help; he was too tough for that. He also mistakenly believed that if he were kind and supportive to himself, he'd lose his competitive edge. As a tough guy, he thought he needed to flagellate himself for every missed financial mark to spur himself on and keep fighting. Instead, he became so deflated he just wanted to give up.

BECOMING AN INNER ALLY MAKES YOU STRONGER

When the going gets tough, what really helps the tough get going is self-compassion. One of the reasons self-compassion is so effective at helping us get back up on our feet is that it transforms our inner voice from an enemy to an ally. Think about it: When you go into battle, what's going to be most helpful? Cutting yourself down and doubting yourself or propping yourself up and supporting yourself?

The research is very clear that self-compassion offers strength and resilience:

+ It helps people cope with divorce or raising special-needs children.

+ It helps people with life-threatening illnesses like cancer.

+ It helps people get through natural disasters like hurricanes.

+ It helps war veterans who have experienced combat get through trauma without being emotionally destroyed by it.

+ It helped people get through the COVID pandemic with less stress and loneliness.

Although it's not as extreme as being at war, many of us feel the stress of our work as if we were in a combat zone. The nonstop demands on our time and energy leave us numb and shell-shocked. To turn the tide of the battle, we have to become our own active ally, using mindfulness, common humanity, and kindness to help us win the war with burnout.

When the going gets tough, the tough get going by offering themselves compassion.

SELF-COMPASSION TOOL 3
A Self-Compassionate Letter for Burnout

One effective way to cultivate compassion for yourself is by writing a compassionate letter to yourself. There are three main ways you can write the letter:

1. Think of an imaginary friend who is unconditionally wise, loving, and compassionate and write a letter to yourself *from the perspective of your friend*.

2. Write a letter *as if you were talking to a dearly beloved friend* who was struggling with the same concerns as you.

3. Write a letter from the compassionate part of yourself to the part of yourself that is struggling.

First, choose the way that you are going to write the letter from the three listed above. Next, write yourself a letter from this perspective that explicitly brings the components of self-compassion (mindfulness, common humanity, and self-kindness) to bear on your experience of burnout.

+ Write a paragraph that mindfully acknowledges the feelings of exhaustion and burnout you're experiencing, validating your struggle.

+ Write a paragraph that acknowledges that your feelings are human and that you are not alone in experiencing burnout.

+ Write a paragraph that expresses kindness, encouragement, warmth, and care for what you're going through.

After writing the letter, you can put it down for a while and then read it later, letting the words support and comfort you when you need it most.

It can take a while to feel comfortable writing to yourself in a compassionate way, but it definitely gets easier with practice. If you especially like writing, you can write a self-compassion letter every night before going to sleep. Research shows that the more you practice self-compassion, the more self-compassionate you will become.

Here's a letter that Isaiah wrote for himself. Isaiah had been a star athlete on his high school football team, and he had a coach who was very kind and supportive. He could tell his coach anything, and his coach would listen patiently and respond in a manner that always made Isaiah feel better. So Isaiah wrote his letter to himself from the perspective of his old coach, using the nickname his coach had given him: Rocketman (because Isaiah was a fast runner and loved Elton John). The three paragraphs in Isaiah's letter reflect the three components of self-compassion.

Hey, Rocketman,

I know how exhausted you are. You're still trying to score a touchdown on every play, and it's wearing you out. You're not sleeping well, and you don't feel like yourself. The energy and optimism that used to lift up the whole team, especially after a loss, is hard to find these days. I know you're struggling. So much responsibility—too much, really.

Remember that starting a business is hard for everyone. There's nothing wrong with you for feeling overwhelmed—it's completely human. You're a person, not a machine. You need a break, too. Anyone in your situation would feel like it's too much.

I really care about you, Rocketman, and I'm sad to see you in this state. But don't give up on yourself or your business just yet. You can make some changes that will help. First of all, you can delegate more responsibility to your team. Give some of your workload to others so they can shoulder part of the burden. Also, remember that it's okay to miss sales targets and fail, because—as I tried to always drill into the team—we learn from failures. Instead of taking it personally, try to learn what went

> *wrong and correct it. That's actually what's going to help you grow your business.*
>
> *Just take it day by day and see how it goes, okay? I believe in you. You'll get through this.*
>
> *Love, Coach*

Isaiah felt funny writing the letter at first, but he put it in the drawer of his nightstand and read it every night for a week. He could feel the compassion in his letter, which allowed him to take it in and even follow his own advice. Isaiah began working shorter hours and giving more responsibility to others. He started seeing disappointing sales figures as learning opportunities rather than failures. Isaiah also recognized that there was a part of himself—a wise and compassionate inner coach—that he could access by thinking of his high school mentor. Isaiah didn't sell his business, and eventually he recovered his dazzling smile.

Self-compassion isn't difficult; we just aren't in the habit of doing it. Luckily, we can draw on our experiences with compassion received from or given to others as a template. If we're mindful of our pain, remember that we aren't alone, and give ourselves kindness and support, we can transform our ability to cope with stress. Misconceptions about self-compassion often stand in our way, however—a topic addressed in the next chapter.

4

IT'S NOT WHAT YOU THINK

Misgivings about Self-Compassion

Even when we feel depleted and exhausted, many of us resist giving ourselves the support and kindness we could really use. In fact, it's precisely when we're reaching total burnout that we may be most likely to reject self-compassion. Because we're so used to giving our all without crumbling, we may blame ourselves for running out of gas and decide that we don't deserve any compassion. Sometimes the harder it becomes to do our work, the harder we are on ourselves.

There's lots of evidence that self-compassion can help us relate better to burnout. But even a mountain of evidence still has to compete with some entrenched cultural misconceptions about this supportive mindset. Dispelling these notions is a good idea since they often block us from benefiting from self-compassion.

MYTHS ABOUT SELF-COMPASSION

Over the years we've observed that people often have mistaken beliefs about what self-compassion is and what it isn't. Do any of the following sound familiar?

- ❏ Self-compassion means wallowing in self-pity.
- ❏ Giving ourselves compassion is selfish.
- ❏ Self-compassion is narcissistic.

- ❏ Self-compassion will make us soft or weak.
- ❏ Self-compassion is self-indulgent.
- ❏ If we're self-compassionate, we'll avoid taking personal responsibility.
- ❏ If we're self-compassionate, we'll lose our drive and motivation to change.

Interestingly, misperceptions like these seem to be pretty universal. We've taught self-compassion around the world, and people everywhere typically check off at least two or three of these misgivings. An example is Giada.

Giada has been working as a public defender for twenty-five years. She represents people charged with crimes ranging from drug possession and shoplifting to theft and murder. The clients assigned to her by the state are poor and often struggle with mental illness or drug addiction. She understands the tough knocks her clients have had in life and strongly believes that every person deserves competent legal counsel whether they can afford it or not, but her clients can be challenging and demanding. She's starting to tune out and is feeling less engaged in her work.

Giada is also beginning to tune out at home—or she wishes she could. Her twenty-year-old son is struggling in community college just as he did in high school, and the minute Giada drags herself in the front door he confronts her with demands for reassurance that he's not going to flunk out. Too often these exchanges call up images of clients who demand reassurance from her that they aren't going to jail. One day after working with a particularly taxing client who took up her whole afternoon and arriving home to her son's vocal worrying about his upcoming exams, Giada lost it and yelled, "WOULD YOU PLEASE GIVE ME A BREAK!" She felt awful and immediately apologized. As she hunched over the kitchen counter trying to prepare dinner, she started to cry silently as she thought about all the stress she was under. But she just shook herself angrily and said internally to stop feeling sorry for herself.

Giada could use a little self-compassion. In fact, her neighbor gave her a book to read about it. But Giada is caught in a trap created by messages she heard growing up. She learned that compassion is only for others. The idea that it could also be for herself just feels "wrong." Her parents were hard workers who were determined to give their children a better life than they had and instilled in her the values of stoicism and self-sacrifice. Giada feared that being compassionate to herself would make her a lazy, self-centered whiner. Giada's skepticism about self-compassion has deep roots, but it also denies her access to a proven solution to burnout.

Giada would probably be more willing to try self-compassion if she knew her misgivings were actually misconceptions: most of the common worries about self-compassion have been disproven by research.

Self-Compassion Is Not Self-Pity

Self-pity may conjure up a picture of curling up in a little ball for days, wailing about how unfair the world is. Or complaining about how much harder you have it than anyone else. You don't want to be that person. Fortunately, self-compassion doesn't ask you to be.

Compassion and pity are quite different. Pity involves looking down on someone and feeling sorry for them. Compassion says "We've all been there." Pity creates separation, and compassion creates connection. It's similar with ourselves. Self-pity isolates us via self-talk like "Poor me" or "Why am I the only one who has to deal with this?" Self-compassion reminds us that everyone struggles at times. Instead of feeling resentful about what we imagine is our uniquely heavy burden, the common humanity component of self-compassion reminds us that others have similar burdens. This gets us out of the rabbit hole of "Why me?" thinking.

Self-pity traps us in the claustrophobic confines of our own head. Self-compassion frees us to see that all humans struggle.

The mindfulness aspect of self-compassion helps to break the cycle of rumination that drives self-pity. It gives us some distance from the repetitive negative thoughts and feelings that only make burnout worse. When we pause for a few breaths and validate our pain ("This moment is really hard") without getting lost in it ("My life is over"), we gain perspective so that we don't exaggerate how bad things are.

Although self-compassion turns kindness inward, it actually reduces self-focus. Research shows that self-compassionate people ruminate less often and are less likely to feel isolated by their difficulties. Having compassion for yourself doesn't mean you wallow in pain. When you remember that you're part of a greater whole and open your heart to the shared human experience of suffering, you're less likely to play a starring role in your own soap opera.

Self-Compassion Is Not Selfish

We sometimes assume caring is a zero-sum game: "I have only five units of compassion, so giving three to myself will leave only two for anyone else." Many of us have gotten the message that it's noble to put others ahead of ourselves, so we use most of our resources to meet others' needs. To use some of those precious resources for ourselves, we believe, would be selfish. Giada certainly got this message from her mother, who never complained about cooking and cleaning and caring for her four children while working almost full-time as a waitress.

But it doesn't work that way. The more compassion we give to ourselves, the more compassion we have available to give to others. Research shows that self-compassionate people are more giving, warm, and loving in their relationships than those who are mean to themselves. They're also more likely to compromise when their own needs conflict with those of others—not putting themselves first or last. Furthermore, self-compassionate people are more likely to give to others authentically—because they want to, not because feel they have to in order to be "good." This authenticity fosters more closeness and intimacy with others. Not only does increasing self-compassion increase feelings of compassion for others, importantly, it allows us to enjoy (rather than resent) caring for others.

Self-Compassion Is Not Narcissistic

A lot of people think that being compassionate toward yourself means building up your ego and enhancing your self-esteem. Self-esteem is an evaluation of self-worth that often comes from feeling special and above average. The self-worth of self-compassion comes from knowing that each of us is a flawed human among flawed human beings, and we're all worthy and valuable. We don't need to feel better than others to feel good about ourselves.

Narcissism says it's all about me. Self-compassion says it's all about us.

The need to feel special and superior leaves us constantly scanning for the next contender who wants to replace us on the pedestal. It's anxiety provoking because, let's face it, there's always going to be someone doing it better. With self-compassion, we don't see competitors; we see comrades—fellow travelers on the bumpy road of life. Research has shown that self-worth derived from self-compassion doesn't depend on comparisons with others. The self-worth of self-compassion is also highly stable over time because it's always there for us, in good times and bad.

Self-Compassion Is Not Wimpy

People often see self-compassion as soft and weak. But don't worry, self-compassion will not turn you into a lump of dough; it's one of the most powerful sources of inner strength, coping, and resilience we have available to us. As we mentioned in the last chapter, research shows that self-compassion fortifies us for the tough times, whether it's caring for a family member who's chronically ill, working at a stressful job, going through a divorce, or fighting for justice in a world teeming with inequities. Being able to support and encourage yourself gives you greater ability to handle challenges and means you'll be less likely to run out of steam.

Studies conducted with combat soldiers, for instance, found that soldiers who were compassionate to themselves after returning to civilian life were less likely to develop posttraumatic stress disorder (PTSD), abuse alcohol, or contemplate suicide as a way to escape their pain. They functioned much better in daily life and were even able to learn and grow from their horrific experiences. And the amount of compassion they gave themselves was a stronger predictor of whether they developed PTSD than how much action they saw. How we relate to ourselves when times are tough—giving ourselves the cold shoulder or a supportive pat—makes all the difference in our ability to cope with life's challenges.

Self-Compassion Is Not Self-Indulgent

A common worry is that self-compassion just means going easy on yourself. "I'll go ahead and hit the snooze button for the seventh time even though I'll be late for that important meeting because—gosh darn it—I'm tired and I deserve it!" We often think self-compassion means choosing what feels good over what's healthy. If you're burned out, sometimes you do need to go easier on yourself to be well. Sometimes you need to pamper yourself and get a massage or take a vacation. But self-indulgence, by definition, means choosing short-term pleasure over long-term harm. If you care about yourself and don't want to suffer, you won't engage in behaviors that harm you in the long run.

Research shows that self-compassion leads to healthy behaviors like eating more nutritious food, exercising, consulting your doctor, and getting more sleep. Just as a compassionate parent doesn't indulge their child because of the harm it might cause, self-compassion spurs us to ask, "What do I need right now to be well?"

Self-Compassion Will Not Let You Off the Hook

Sometimes people think that having compassion for their mistakes and failures means not taking responsibility for misdeeds. While it's true that with self-compassion you don't mercilessly attack yourself when you recognize you've caused harm, paradoxically, this allows you to take greater personal responsibility for what you've done. Think about it. If you know that acknowledging you've done something wrong or hurtful means blasting yourself with harsh criticism, your subconscious will do everything in its power to distort events and blame someone else. The consequences of owning up to the truth are just too great. With self-compassion, it's safe to acknowledge you've screwed up. It's human. It happens to everyone from time to time.

Research shows that self-compassion doesn't reduce guilt (feeling bad about harming someone), but it does reduce shame (feeling bad about yourself for harming someone). It also shows that people who are helped to have compassion for past harm are more likely to take personal responsibility for their actions, apologize, and try to repair the situation.

Self-Compassion Will Not Undermine Your Motivation

Call it your drive, your edge, or your motivation, giving yourself compassion won't make you stop trying your hardest. There's little risk of turning into a complacent, lazy ne'er-do-well. But many people don't realize this. Whether it's work productivity, athletics, raising kids, or studying for exams, we have reams of research evidence that beating ourselves up doesn't work nearly as well for motivating change as warmth, validation, and encouragement.

Think back to the best boss you ever had. Did the person motivate you to do your best by abusing you? Fear is a strong motivator, but not for long; you probably put distance between a bad boss and yourself as soon as you could. That boss may have also undermined your confidence to the point that you thought of giving up that line of work altogether. A boss who had high expectations but also believed in you and encouraged you and helped you to learn from your mistakes was probably much more effective. In fact, the ability to have compassion for our failures without taking them personally is precisely what allows us to pick ourselves up and try again (more about self-compassionate motivation in Chapter 18).

TAKING A LEAP INTO SELF-COMPASSION

Because most cultures don't encourage self-compassion and are even downright suspicious of it, we don't get many messages that help us adopt this supportive stance. When we're already feeling overwhelmed and burned out, it can be especially hard to remember to be self-compassionate. For this reason, it's worth considering ways to make it easier to remember to be self-compassionate in your daily life.

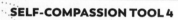

SELF-COMPASSION TOOL 4
Craft a Self-Compassion Reminder

As with all new habits, you need to practice the new habit of self-compassion repeatedly to replace your old habit of self-criticism. Taking the time to craft simple self-compassion practice reminders can help.

Try these:

+ Tie a ribbon around your wrist as a reminder to use self-compassion when you're really stressed. Pick your favorite color as a gesture of self-kindness.

+ Tape a self-compassionate message on your bathroom mirror so you see it before work. A worn-out doctor wrote, "You got this—and if you don't, I'm still here for you."

+ Set your phone or computer opening screen to an encouraging image. Thousands of GIFs (animated images) are available online, such as a heart inscribed with the words "Be Kind to Yourself!" Or you can use a picture that symbolizes self-compassion. A father working two jobs to support his family used a photo of himself at his favorite beach at sunset to remind himself that he is worthy of care.

+ Write little messages about self-compassion on sticky notes and put them in places you'll see throughout the day: you can put "Remember mindfulness, common humanity, and self-kindness" in your desk drawer or "You deserve self-compassion" on your coffee maker or "It's okay to be imperfect" on your refrigerator. Those sticky notes have to be good for something, right?

+ Set a daily pop-up reminder on your phone to do a short compassion practice, like the tender self-compassion break (see Chapter 6).

We can't always depend on others to provide us with compassion when we need it. But we have what we need to start to emerge from burnout in our own hearts: the ability to accept and soothe our own pain with tender self-compassion and the strength to defend our well-being with fierce self-compassion. Knowing that research has debunked myths about self-compassion can encourage us to dismiss erroneous worries that might deter us.

After more encouragement from her neighbor, Giada decided to give self-compassion a try. It didn't come naturally to her, so she put little yellow sticky notes on her file cabinet at work and all around her home with kind messages like "Just take it one step at a time," "You're only human," "It's okay to take a break," "It's okay to say no," and "The more compassion you give yourself the more you'll have available to give others." After a while she started to experience little moments of self-compassion throughout her day. At work when she started to feel overwhelmed with a client, she would tell herself that it was only natural to feel that way. When she got home and her son rattled off his worries and insecurities, she acknowledged that it was hard to confront such a barrage of negativity after a hard day's work. She was doing the best she could. These little moments of self-kindness then gave her the emotional space needed to have compassion for her son, who was also trying his best to cope in an academic system he found challenging. With practice, her constant shame and anxiety started to be replaced by a more supportive inner voice saying that she was okay and that everything was going to be okay. Eventually, she found that her resentment and feelings of disconnection began to ease.

Clearing up misconceptions about self-compassion reduces barriers we may have toward adopting this caring approach. However, human physiology and our instinctive way of responding to stress also make self-compassion difficult. The next chapter explores the physiology of stress and care and how being compassionate to ourselves can change the way the nervous system reacts to stressful circumstances.

5

YOUR BODY KNOWS

The Physiology of Stress and Care

Your body knows when you're burned out. Push it too hard and it rebels, maybe with a pounding headache, crushing fatigue, or a roiling stomach. Sometimes all three. When these and other physical symptoms occur every day, you might wonder how your own body can turn on you so cruelly when you need it more than ever to get things done.

It may be hard to believe right now, but your body is trying to protect you. Since the appearance of humans on the planet, our bodies have been relying on an exquisite self-preservation mechanism to keep us moving along. Here's how it works.

THE PHYSIOLOGY OF STRESS

You've probably been the beneficiary of this protective mechanism in its most primitive form, maybe when you've gotten caught in a sudden storm: your sense of touch tells you the temperature has dropped and the wind has picked up . . . your ears hear the rumble of thunder . . . you see a flash of lightning and hear a loud crack. This all happens in an instant. Without thinking, you run for cover, narrowly escaping being conked on the head by a falling tree limb.

What's at work in moments like these is the sympathetic nervous system, otherwise known as the *threat-defense system*. It's also sometimes referred to as the *fight/flight/freeze response* for the options it gives us to save our lives in an emergency. When our senses perceive danger, this system readies the body to fight off a hungry predator, flee from a car barreling straight at us, or freeze and stand stock-still either to escape notice or to give the prefrontal cortex a moment to come up with the best lifesaving strategy. It's partly thanks to this self-preservation system that the species *Homo sapiens* has survived for hundreds of thousands of years.

Work stress can also trigger the threat-defense system, whether we're protecting ourselves or others. A critical care nurse rushes to a patient's side as the monitors signal trouble. A safari guide hushes and stills their group as they unexpectedly come across a bull elephant in the bush. A wounded soldier runs with a wounded comrade twice her weight on her back as they come under enemy attack.

Ahmed is a day trader who invests for many loyal customers. He watches the ups and downs of the market like a hawk, ready to buy or sell at a moment's notice. Even though he knows the market is unstable, he reacts to every price drop as if he were being bombarded with artillery. Usually, he responds with skill and precision. But after fifteen years of trading, he's so tightly wound that he can't sleep through the night, fearful of what the markets will be doing when he wakes up. The constant stress is starting to make Ahmed irritable at home as well as work, and he's losing his self-confidence. His trading acumen is slowly becoming impaired, and he's not making the smart investments he used to.

For traders like Ahmed, the fight/flight/freeze response is like the fuel injection system in a Ferrari: no speed without it. But problems arise when this response drives us all the time, including when we aren't actually threatened. And most of the common threats we face in modern daily life aren't matters of life and death.

STRESS IN MODERN LIFE

Unlike our distant ancestors, we're not too likely to run into a hungry tiger prowling for its dinner. We are, however, vulnerable to a million different modern stressors. Stress is defined as the physical, mental, or emotional tension caused by demanding situations and adverse events that throw us out of our usual equilibrium. That covers a lot of territory, especially where our most important endeavors are concerned. We feel threatened by impossible deadlines, short staffing, heartless leadership. Even the tasks we take on with love and devotion, like caring for a chronically ill child, start to deplete our resources, and then exhaustion or frustration is added to the other stressors involved in our work.

The threat-defense system doesn't realize we're not about to get eaten alive. All it knows is that when we feel threatened, its job is to be our internal first responder. This is helpful when we're trying to pull an all-nighter to file a grant proposal on time or make a last push to the finish line in an important race. Problems build, however, when instead of a one-and-done event, multiple stressors come at us all day long. The system becomes hypervigilant and starts kicking in unnecessarily. It sends Ahmed flying across the kitchen table to catch a dropped piece of toast, for instance, knocking into his kids along the way, in the same manner it kicks him into action to make a trade.

The threat-defense system is hardwired to protect us from life-endangering events, but it often overreacts to everyday stressors.

The types of stressors we live with today typically don't let up. Sales goals, a mobbed ER, crazy competition in our marketplace, money problems, and daily caregiving make constant demands on our resources. This means our threat-defense system is turned on more than it's turned off. We can feel as if we're always crouched in the starting blocks, ready to sprint at a moment's notice. Pretty soon we're suffering from chronic stress, and from there it's just a hop, a skip, and a jump to burnout.

HOW CHRONIC STRESS WEARS THE BODY DOWN

We have plenty of scientific data on the damage that chronic stress can do. The threat-defense system releases the hormones adrenaline and cortisol into our blood vessels to set off changes to bodily functions that prepare us to fight, flee, or freeze. Our heart rate and breathing speed up so we can pound hard or run fast. Functions like digestion that don't contribute to self-defense slow down. Our airways widen, and our heart rate increases to send extra oxygen to our muscles and to increase alertness. Extra fuel in the form of stored glucose gets sent to the body parts that we need most in an emergency, and our senses get sharper too.

Getting revved up like this is extremely effective in the short term, in small doses. But when our heart rate and blood pressure are elevated over the long term, or too frequently, our cardiovascular system is strained. We become exhausted and depleted—that is, we burn out—and our health suffers.

No wonder it sometimes feels as if your body is your enemy. Unabated stress leaves you suffering the effects of an overzealous but well-meaning threat-defense system and can lead to all sorts of health problems.

WHEN THE FIGHT/FLIGHT/FREEZE RESPONSE TURNS INWARD

But here's where things get really dicey: many of our modern-day threats are not to our survival but to our self-worth and sense of competence. When we feel broken and overwhelmed, we often assume it's because we're not doing enough, or not doing it right, or that there is something wrong with us. We start seeing our own inadequacy as the biggest danger we face, so what do we do? We turn the threat-defense system on ourselves in an effort to find safety.

If we're the threat that needs to be defended against, the best approach is to fix ourselves, right? If we can just get our act together and try harder, we'll solve our problems and be safe. So we fight ourselves and mentally beat ourselves up for not being more competent. This helps us feel safe because we think self-criticism will help us change for the better. We then flee into feelings of shame and isolate ourselves, helping us feel safe because we feel less exposed to the judgments of others. Finally, we freeze and ruminate on our horrible selves or lives. This helps us feel safe because we believe if we remain motionless and

---

Is your health being affected by chronic stress in any of these ways?

- ❑ Changes in appetite and eating habits
- ❑ Digestive problems such as ulcers or acid reflux
- ❑ Increased drinking or drug use
- ❑ Lowered sexual desire or functioning
- ❑ Muscle aches and pains
- ❑ High blood pressure

think hard enough we'll figure out how to escape our problems. Sadly, instead of helping ourselves, we're just kicking ourselves when we're down and making it harder to get up.

Ahmed often falls into this trap. He started hanging out in his basement man cave after work in the hope of protecting his young kids from his moody outbursts. There he could rage at the athletes in whatever game he was watching instead of at his family. But when he emerges he still sometimes snaps at his kids, and when he sees the wounded looks on their faces, he berates himself for being a bad dad *and* a failing trader. Ahmed feels stuck in shame and retreats even further into his basement; his wife sometimes even brings him dinner down there.

Unfortunately, turning the threat-defense system inward just makes things a thousand times worse. How can we possibly feel safe when we're treating ourselves as if we're both the predator and the prey? Luckily for us, we have another physiological system that evolved to help human beings survive: the care system.

THE CARE SYSTEM TO THE RESCUE

An important way for humans to feel safe is through feelings of warmth and connection. The care system (sometimes called the attachment system) refers to the mental and emotional bonds that arise when we care for others or are cared for by others. It evolved to ensure that parents would look after their offspring and group members would look after each other, ensuring the survival of the species. The care system releases oxytocin (known as the *love hormone*) and endorphins (our natural, soothing painkillers), helping us feel comforted and calm. It also stimulates the parasympathetic nervous system, often known as the *rest-and-digest system*, which counteracts sympathetic arousal. After the need for self-defense has eased off, our levels of cortisol and adrenaline drop, our heart rate and blood pressure lower, our digestion gets back online, and we generally chill out. We start to feel relaxed, open, and safe.

The threat-defense and care systems work together toward the perpetuation of our species. The first protects us from whatever wants to kill us, and the second promotes the continuation of our genetic line. The threat-defense system evolved primarily for self-preservation, and the care system evolved primarily for other-preservation. That's why it feels more natural to criticize ourselves and be compassionate to others. It also explains why we use the threat-defense system more quickly and easily than the care system, given that our most basic need is to stay alive. When we can't meet a deadline, for instance, we sense danger, so we instinctually respond with fight/flight/freeze turned inward. When a good friend can't meet a deadline, we don't feel personally threatened, so instead we can be warm and supportive.

In many ways, we can think of self-compassion as the process of turning the care system inward in response to threat. It doesn't feel entirely natural, but our bodies don't know the difference.

The threat-defense system evolved to protect us and the care system to protect others; that's why we instinctually criticize ourselves but are compassionate to others.

Research shows that self-compassion activates the parasympathetic nervous system (linked to the care system) and deactivates the sympathetic nervous system (linked to the threat-defense system). For example, self-compassion increases heart rate variability, an indicator of parasympathetic activity and of how responsive and flexible the heart is to changing conditions. Self-compassion also decreases cortisol and stress-related markers such as inflammation. This difference in nervous system response leads to greater health: self-compassionate people have better immune function because their sympathetic system isn't constantly in overdrive. They also sleep better, which allows the body to recover from stress.

Self-compassion helps us respond better psychologically and emotionally to stressors so they're less likely to overwhelm us, and in fact research shows that self-compassion is linked to lower perceptions of stress. We feel safer when stressed because we have our own back, which means that the stress doesn't feel like life and death. We see it with greater balance and perspective. Self-compassion also alters the way we respond to internal threats in the form of feelings of incompetence or low self-worth. We respond with care rather than fight/flight/freeze, meaning we aren't so self-critical, don't feel so isolated, and ruminate less on our stress. We're more accepting of our human imperfections and use kindness to encourage adaptation and change.

But how do we tap into the care system when stressed, especially since it feels more natural and instinctual to go into threat-defense mode? There's a hack we can use: physical touch. The body is closely wired to our autonomic nervous system and can change our physiological responses more quickly than our thoughts. Even before infants learn to speak, parents demonstrate compassion to their infants by holding and rocking them. They may coo or sing quietly and soothingly. This makes the baby feel calm and safe even though they have no idea what their parents are saying. By using our bodies as a vehicle for the expression of compassion, we can help ourselves tap into the care system even if our minds aren't yet ready to go there. This helps to reverse the physiological effects of an overactive threat-defense response.

THE POWER OF TOUCH

Have you ever seen someone in distress standing with hands grasping their upper arms as if they're hugging themselves, gently swaying back and forth? Some of us instinctually turn to our bodies for comfort when under stress. Is there something you turn to when stressed out? Some people love the feeling of being immersed in a warm, fragrant bath, feeling hot tea slip down their throat, or having a light massage. Even letting the sun warm your skin can have a similar effect. The most direct way to physically tap into the parasympathetic nervous system, however, is through soothing and supportive touch. One study showed that soothing self-touch such as placing a hand on your own heart reduces cortisol in much the same way as the supportive touch of another.

When you receive worrying news or feel inadequate or are so exhausted you can't take another step, you can give yourself compassion physically. You can feel the warmth of your own hands on your body, activating the care system and helping you feel safer. This will help calm the feelings of stress fueling your burnout.

SELF-COMPASSION TOOL 5
Supportive Touch

It's important to identify a type of touch that you find supportive. Sometimes our touch has a gentle, tender quality that can help soothe and calm us. But touch can also have a fierce empowering quality that provides strength and courage. Explore the possibilities in the following list and come up with your own variations until you hit on something that truly helps you feel safe in the moment. And if any type of touch makes you feel uncomfortable, stop and try something else. Everyone responds differently. Stick with each for about ten seconds and note how you react during that time.

Supportive Touch

+ Put one or both hands over your heart.
+ Put one fist on your heart (symbolizing strength), then cover it with the other hand.
+ Put one hand on your heart and one on your stomach.
+ Put one or both hands on your solar plexus (between your navel and ribcage).
+ Put one hand on your cheek or cradle your face in your hands.
+ Plant your hands strongly on your hips (like Wonder Woman).
+ Squeeze one hand with the other.
+ Give yourself a hug and rock back and forth.

Optional: Supportive Sounds. Some people find it helpful to add in language or sounds to supportive touch; see the examples in the following list.

Supportive Sounds

+ Whisper a kind message: "You've got this." "I won't abandon you."
+ Make noises that feel good to you, like "awwww" or "ohhhh."
+ Hum or sing a song that you find calming, encouraging, or uplifting.
+ Exhale through pursed lips, like a weightlifter.

Once you think you've found one or two types of touch that make you feel safe and cared for, take them into the real world and test them out. Like the other tools and strategies in this book, supportive touch can be used anywhere, anytime. A nurse at a patient's bedside can discreetly grasp one hand with the other to offer herself warmth. If you read something disturbing on your computer, you can cradle your face in your hands to minimize the shock. You can hum a calming tune to yourself while walking to a meeting you're nervous about. If touching your own body is uncomfortable, try hugging a favorite soft pillow or wrapping yourself in a thick, warm blanket.

Ahmed felt a bit embarrassed to try supportive touch at first. What if someone saw him? But when he was sure no one was watching, he tried gently rubbing his arms as an expression of kindness to himself. On other occasions, Ahmed sang himself a lullaby in Arabic that his grandmother used to sing to him as a child. No one knew what he was doing, but it made a big difference.

Soothing and supportive self-touch can help us turn down the volume on the threat-defense system and turn it up on the care system. Another way to activate the care system is through the power of language. The next chapter will explore further how words, especially the *tone* of our words, can be used to activate tender self-compassion.

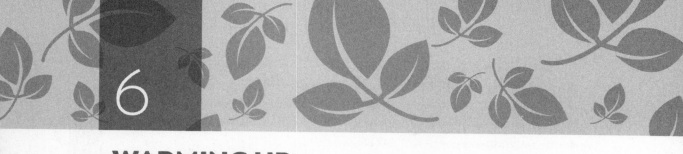

6

WARMING UP THE CONVERSATION

Tender Acceptance

When we hit the wall of burnout, we may be overcome with emotion—feeling sad, worthless, angry, frustrated, resentful, defeated, empty, or numb—and then rail against the deluge, hoping that fighting our feelings will make them go away. Maybe we give ourselves hell for being weak and incompetent, then withdraw into a cave like a wounded animal, hiding in shame. As we discussed in the last chapter, we're hardwired to go into fight/flight/freeze (aka *freakout*) mode when stressed, and when the "threat" comes from inside us as negative thoughts and feelings, we're likely to turn on ourselves. But when we tap into our natural capacity for care and connection, things go much better.

WARMING THINGS UP

Self-compassion has two main expressions: tender acceptance and fierce action. The healing balm of tender self-compassion is especially helpful when dealing with the feelings of inadequacy and despair linked to burnout. Tender self-compassion promotes resilience and recovery, which is exactly what we need when we're burned out. We can tap into it by shifting the language and tone of our inner voice so that it's warm and friendly rather than cold and demeaning toward ourselves.

You know the power of tenderness. Maybe you've seen a toddler fall and start wailing, only to stop crying the moment Dad scoops them up. Or perhaps you've gazed into the eyes of a friend who'd suffered a loss, and witnessed how they felt comforted by your visual embrace. Our natural response tends to be gentle rather than harsh when someone we care about is suffering. Can you imagine telling a valued coworker who was trembling from exhaustion at the end of a twelve-hour shift to stop being such a wuss? Probably not. You're more likely to say "Poor thing, please sit down. It's been crazy around here. Can I get you anything?" Yet when the shoe is on the other foot—when *we're* struggling or feel broken—tenderness doesn't come quite so easily.

Jada had to grow up fast when her mother passed away five years ago. She's now twenty-four years old and the primary caretaker of her fourteen-year-old brother, Dion, who has cerebral palsy. Jada wakes up at dawn every morning, prepares Dion's lunch, helps him get ready for school, and puts him on the bus at 7:00 A.M. Then she goes to work as the assistant manager of a computer store from 7:30 A.M. to 4:00 P.M. and is back in time to help Dion get off the bus. Jada fixes dinner for them both and then helps Dion bathe. From 7:30 P.M. to 11:30 P.M. Jada works a second job from home, troubleshooting for an internet service provider. Weekends are better, but Jada still needs to take Dion to his appointments and manage the household. The routine is wearing Jada down with no end in sight.

Jada is bitter about the raw deal she got—robbed of her mother and also her own carefree youth. But she doesn't want to wallow in self-pity. She thinks she just has to be tough and push through. After all, at least she's physically healthy, unlike Dion. Her mother was an incredibly strong woman and never complained, somehow managing to keep a smile on her face no matter how difficult things were. Jada knows her mother would want her to step up to the plate. Whenever she starts to feel sad or hopeless, Jada metaphorically shakes herself and says, "Snap out of it, you big baby! Complaining helps no one."

HOW ARE YOU RELATING TO YOURSELF?

Tender self-compassion gives us the capacity to *be with* ourselves just as we are, even if we're a tattered, burned-out mess. It has the quality of a loving parent relating to a newborn child. It doesn't matter if the infant is crying uncontrollably or just pooped in their diaper. Somehow most parents manage to love their children regardless. With tender self-compassion, we adopt a similar attitude toward ourselves. Just as it's possible to hold a cranky baby, we can hold ourselves in the middle of difficult feelings like frustration, anger, shame, or despair so that we don't feel so overwhelmed.

Importantly, with tender self-compassion we focus less on what's happening and more on how we're *relating* to what's happening. Rather than being lost in or consumed by feelings of burnout, we settle into an attitude of care and concern toward ourselves simply *because* we're burned out. Our attention shifts from the content of our experience to the quality of how we're holding it. Is my heart open or closed? Am I accepting myself as I am or judging and criticizing myself? Am I being helpful or making things worse? Is my inner dialogue warm or cold? When we relate to our experience of burnout with tender acceptance, we start to feel calmer yet also energized because we feel safe and cared for. Tender self-compassion feels good without requiring us to cover up or deny that burnout feels bad.

> **Tender self-compassion helps us focus less on what's happening and more on how we're relating to what's happening.**

TRY A LITTLE TENDERNESS

When you're burned out, beating yourself up in an attempt to get over it only wears you down further. Tender self-compassion can help you heal from burnout by offering yourself comfort, soothing, and validation.

- **Comfort** means responding to our *emotional* needs in a compassionate manner. What emotions are you feeling? Hurt? Fear? Loneliness? Shame? And what do you need when you feel like that? If you feel sad, maybe you need to listen to some music or walk in the woods? If you're frightened, maybe you need to talk with a friend? Comfort usually has a tender quality. Think of how you respond to a close colleague who is really upset by a traumatic work experience. You probably say something like "I'm so sorry. Are you okay? I'm right here for you." When you're distressed because you're burned out, what words of comfort can you offer yourself? Sometimes a warm nod of recognition is all that's needed.

- **Soothing** refers to our *physical* needs—quieting the overstressed body. When you're burned out, your body has probably been pushed to the limit, not just by exhaustion on the job but also from not eating or sleeping well. To soothe yourself physically, you might want to take a rest, settle into a warm bath, get a massage, or drink a cup of tea. You can also give yourself supportive touch (see Chapter 5), such as tenderly placing a hand over your heart or another body part that is holding stress.

- **Validation** is the process of understanding and honoring the pain of burnout. It's *relational*, and in the case of self-compassion, it's how we relate to ourselves. We often subtly assume that we shouldn't feel so exhausted; that there's something wrong with us for feeling this way. Validating the pain acknowledges that you're struggling and that you're fully human for doing so. *Of course* you're burned out given everything you've been dealing with. Anyone would feel this way in similar circumstances. It's important to recognize and name your distress in a caring way to begin to work with it.

WE'RE ALL DOING THE BEST WE CAN

Giving ourselves tender acceptance for being burned out is an acknowledgment that we're doing the best we can right now. As human beings we have limited resources and coping skills, we just can't do everything, and we certainly can't do everything *right*. One reason we criticize ourselves for being burned out or inadequate is that it gives us the illusion of control. Some part of us believes it's possible to be Hercules. We fall into the trap of thinking "If I just tried a little harder or were stronger or smarter or [fill in the blank], I could get the job done." Somehow this seems safer than recognizing the truth—the task is bigger than we are.

Jada felt overwhelmed by her responsibility for Dion, but acknowledging her limitations seemed even more overwhelming. Behind her admirable efforts to meet her responsibilities, Jada was haunted by shame—shame for not being as strong as her mother was. Her plight would have been much more bearable if she knew how to practice tender self-compassion, especially by tapping into its three essential components.

> **Sometimes acknowledging our limitations is hard because it means giving up our sense of control over an uncontrollable situation.**

LOVING, CONNECTED PRESENCE

The three core components of self-compassion—mindfulness, common humanity, and self-kindness—take a particular form when used to alleviate suffering through tender acceptance: *loving, connected presence.*

Mindfulness: Being Present

The first step of a mindful response to burnout is to turn toward and stay present with our discomfort. Part of us may want to stick our head in the sand and pretend that our situation isn't so bad. Or we may get hijacked by our emotions and lose perspective on them. All we see is that the sky is dark with storm clouds. Mindful presence avoids both of these extremes. We're aware of our feelings—hopelessness, despair, anger, exhaustion—but we don't fixate on them. We accept how bad burnout feels without denying or fighting reality.

Imagine that a good friend called you to share a difficult marital issue. To be mindfully present, you'd first have to answer the phone and then carefully listen to what your friend had to share. If you didn't take the call, or if you talked over your friend, giving unsolicited advice, your friend wouldn't feel seen or heard. Similarly, in the relationship we have with ourselves, we need to pick up the phone and listen compassionately to ourselves. The experience of burnout is real, and it deserves our attention. (We'll go more deeply into how to be mindfully present in Chapter 8.)

Common Humanity: Feeling Connected to Others

When you hit the wall of burnout, you're likely to feel isolated and alone. In fact, one of the symptoms of burnout is the tendency to disengage from social life due to exhaustion and disillusionment. It's also not uncommon to assume that everyone but you is coping just fine with workplace stress and thus feel emotionally isolated even when among other people. The truth is that your experience of burnout connects you to millions of other people who are also burned out, including other readers of this book.

Professional and family caregivers everywhere are being worked to the bone. The world is full of demanding employers and unfair workplace practices. Stress is the norm, not the exception. Feeling your connection to other people who are struggling as you are can be a comfort in and of itself. You're a human being living in a human world! Superheroes and relaxed paradises are not real. We all run into our limitations as struggling cohabitants of planet Earth.

And of course, if you examine the reasons you're burned out, you'll find they stem from the coming together of complex causes and conditions—your workplace environment, the larger culture, politics, economics, your genetic predisposition to react to stress, your early family upbringing—most of which are completely out of your control. More interconnected causes and conditions exist than you could possibly identify. Recognizing that truth helps you remember that you are part of a larger whole.

Kindness: Giving Yourself Love

The element of kindness in self-compassion has a loving, nurturing quality when we practice tender acceptance. It's wise and empathic. We treat ourselves with the same warmth and goodwill that we naturally show to those we care about. Let's say your nephew is a nurse and he was upset one day because he forgot to ask a patient an important intake question. You might say something like "Hey, I know you feel bad, but mistakes like this happen. It's not the end of the world; you can call the patient to follow up. You had people lined up back-to-back and were too busy to think straight." This outpouring of support would feel good to both you and your nephew.

An amazing thing about adopting a warm and caring attitude toward our experience of burnout is that it becomes an opportunity to both give and receive love—from ourselves to ourselves. As we learn to become more comfortable with the voice of self-kindness, our ability to love grows stronger. It doesn't have preconditions or require us to fix ourselves or our lives, because love can hold everything.

Want to give tender self-compassion a try and see how it impacts your experience of burnout? The following tool can be used on or off the job.

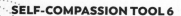

SELF-COMPASSION TOOL 6
Tender Self-Compassion Break

The self-compassion break is one the most popular practices from the MSC program. It intentionally calls in the three components of self-compassion and applies them to our distress. This self-compassion break is designed to evoke tender self-compassion for burnout, and in later chapters the practice will be tailored to evoke different forms of fierce self-compassion.

+ Please sit or lie down in a way that makes you feel comfortable and relaxed.

+ Bring to mind an aspect of burnout that is challenging you right now, especially one that calls for kindness, warmth, or self-acceptance. For example, maybe you're feeling inadequate, drained, depleted, hopeless, or numb. (Don't focus on an injustice, please, which would call for more fierce self-compassion.) Also, please choose a difficulty that isn't overwhelming, so you won't get derailed during this practice.

+ As you think about this burnout experience, allow yourself to feel the stress or discomfort that arises in your body. Where do you feel the most discomfort? See if you can allow the experience to be there, if only for a moment, knowing that's how burnout feels.

+ There are three phrases that you can say to yourself—silently or out loud—that are designed to bring loving, connected presence to your experience of burnout. Although specific words will be suggested, the goal is to find language that works best for you.

+ The first phrase is meant to help you be *mindfully* present with the pain of burnout. Try saying to yourself, slowly and calmly, "This is a moment of suffering." If this language doesn't feel quite right, see if you can come up with some other way of expressing this message, such as "This is hard," "I feel so stressed and exhausted," or "I'm really hurting."

✦ The second phrase is designed to remind you of your *common humanity*. Try saying to yourself, "Burnout is a part of life." Other options are "I'm not alone," "We all face stress in our lives," or "This is how it feels when a person is burned out."

✦ Now, put your hands over your heart, or any place on your body that feels soothing, feeling the warmth and gentle touch of your hands.

✦ The third phrase calls in the power of *love* and *kindness*. Try saying with tenderness, "May I be kind to myself in this moment." Other options might be "May I accept myself as I am," "May I be understanding and patient with myself," or "I'm here for you." If it feels comfortable, you can even try saying, "I love you."

✦ If you're having difficulty finding the right words, imagine that a dear friend was having the same experience you are. What would you say to that person, heart to heart, to soothe and comfort them? Can you offer the same message to yourself?

✦ Before you end this practice, please take a moment to notice how you feel in your body, allowing your experience to be just as it is, and allowing yourself to be just as you are, right here and right now, if only for this one moment.

Jada had heard about the self-compassion break on a podcast. Although it made her a bit uncomfortable, Jada decided to give it a try the next time she felt overwhelmed while caring for Dion. One evening as Jada was helping him bathe, the soap slipped through her fingers and slid under the bathroom vanity and she banged her head as she tried to capture the escapee. As Jada sat on the floor, she felt an urge to sob start to well up. She told Dion she needed a minute and ran into her bedroom to cry. When her sobbing subsided, Jada remembered the self-compassion break.

First, she brought in mindfulness and said to herself, "I'm a mess. I hurt so much. There's nothing about this situation that doesn't hurt." Instead of hiding from feeling overwhelmed, Jada began to turn toward and face her predicament.

Then she told herself that she was probably not the only person in a difficult caregiving situation. Not everyone had a brother with cerebral palsy, but they might have a family member with cancer, mental illness, or some other disability. Caring for someone with high needs was surely overwhelming for everyone at times. "I guess I'm not alone," Jada said to herself.

Jada then put both hands over her pounding heart. Her hands felt warm and solid. She just left them there because it felt good. Jada tried to say a few words of kindness to herself, but nothing came out, so she imagined what her mother would say to her. "I'm so sorry you're going through this, sweetheart. I know how hard it is. Just do the best you can and take it one day at a time. I'm here for you." It worked for Jada to say those exact words to herself. There was some grief in the fact that her mother couldn't be there for her because she had passed, but also some comfort in knowing that Jada could be there for herself. The hammer pounding in her heart started feeling more like a gentle drumbeat. About five minutes later, feeling much calmer, Jada returned to helping Dion wash himself.

This first experience with the self-compassion break encouraged Jada to use the formula again the next time she felt overwhelmed. Over the coming months, Jada noticed she wasn't so cold toward herself, and she also didn't go into overwhelm quite so often. She still felt sad and hopeless sometimes, but there was another voice, a loving and kind voice that reminded her of her mother's. A voice that expressed care and concern and helped her feel supported. It made her situation a bit easier to bear. She knew she was going to be okay, as long as she just took it day by day.

When it seems like burnout has gotten the best of us and we don't know what to do, a good place to start is with tender self-compassion. We can be warm and kind to ourselves simply *because* of the state we're in, without preconditions. Tender self-compassion reverses our tendency to beat ourselves up when things go wrong, and it taps the healing resources of care and connection. However, if we aren't used to opening our hearts with self-compassion, the very act of doing so can be uncomfortable, even scary. The next chapter explores this phenomenon—backdraft—and describes how to harness it to help alleviate burnout.

7

WHEN SELF-COMPASSION FEELS BAD

Working with Backdraft

A moment of compassion is usually a welcome relief. Speaking kindly to yourself when you're upset, or using supportive touch, can be a huge help. But receiving compassion doesn't *always* feel good. Have you ever felt uncomfortable when someone said something kind or complimentary to you? Does it feel weird to say something nice to yourself such as "You're okay just as you are"? If so, you're in good company.

Ben is a high-functioning kind of guy. He has a successful home renovation business that receives top ratings on Yelp and Google. But it's a struggle to keep his customers satisfied. Clients often get angry when renovation projects are stalled while he waits for the right tradespeople to become available. And when his subcontractors mess up, he's held responsible. Ben's evenings and weekends are typically spent resolving problems and arranging logistics—that is, when Ben doesn't have a splitting headache.

Ben's doctor told him he needed to take at least one day off a week because the stress was "messing with his brain" (Ben's words, not his doctor's), but when he did so, he felt like a slacker. Ben was also merciless when he got something wrong on a job, calling himself a "stupid idiot" and worse. His partner, Sybil, had taken a self-compassion course as part of an employee wellness program and realized that Ben needed to be kinder to himself. She thought she would teach him a simple practice like putting his hands on his heart. As soon as Ben lifted his hands to his chest, however, he became agitated and uncomfortable. Self-compassion just seemed to make him feel worse.

When we practice self-compassion, sometimes we feel good, sometimes we feel bad, and sometimes we feel nothing at all. All these reactions are completely normal and part of healing. However, it might be confusing to feel bad after offering yourself compassion. After all, no one starts to practice self-compassion to feel *worse*! If you feel worse, you're likely to think you did something wrong or that self-compassion isn't right for you.

There's a word for the distress that arises when we offer ourselves compassion—"backdraft." *Backdraft* is a firefighting term. It refers to how a fire in an enclosed room intensifies when oxygen is introduced rapidly through an open door or window. Well, the same thing can happen when the doors of our hearts open with self-compassion. Our hearts hold a lot of pain, often from old wounds that we've pushed aside so we can function in our daily lives. When we practice self-compassion and the door of the heart opens, the love goes in and the pain comes out.

If you're experiencing burnout, chances are you've been shutting out emotional pain. When you're kind to yourself, the feelings you've been pushing aside may start to emerge. These feelings are not *caused* by self-compassion; they're being *uncovered*. That's a good thing because you can see them and begin to heal them.

Why does backdraft occur? Because we can only know anything through contrast. We know hot because we know cold. We know light because we also know dark. There's a saying "Love reveals everything unlike itself." If I say to myself, "May I accept myself just as I am," chances are I'll start thinking about my unacceptable qualities or times when others have treated me as if I were unacceptable. This happens naturally, but as you can imagine, those memories are not fun.

In Ben's case, he didn't get as far as putting his hands on his chest, let alone saying kind words to himself. A self-compassionate act like taking a break from work was enough to trigger backdraft. As a child, Ben suffered from undiagnosed attention-deficit/hyperactivity disorder. His father was highly critical of Ben's efforts at school and would often shame him in front of others. In adulthood, although Ben found work that suited his temperament and he was successful, in the back of his mind he was still a "loser" and an "idiot." When Sybil expressed compassion for him, Ben felt anxious. His younger, "loser" self was lurking just beneath the surface, threatening to break through.

What would it take for Ben to be more self-compassionate? He would need to be open to what self-compassion stirred up. At the moment, however, Ben was unable to do that. In this case, the next step is to become *curious* about backdraft.

RECOGNIZING BACKDRAFT

Has backdraft ever come up when you tried to give yourself compassion? Maybe an old self-doubt popped up, or a difficult emotion, or you became physically restless?

When we start to practice self-compassion, old traumas, big and small, can reveal themselves, as if they were waiting for a time when we had the resources to deal with them. For example, you might still be carrying the hurt of being dumped by an old flame, and when you start being compassionate with yourself, you could start thinking about the heartbreak for the first time in years.

If you're curious about backdraft and are wondering what might turn up for you, consider the following questions:

- What gets in the way of your being more self-compassionate?
- What thoughts and feelings are you afraid might come up?
- What are your worries about how self-compassion could impact your life?

Backdraft comes in many forms:

✦ **Mentally,** you might start criticizing yourself, thinking "I'm a mess," "I'm a failure," "I'm worthless."

✦ **Emotionally,** you could suddenly feel shame or guilt, sadness or grief, fear or anxiety, anger or irritation.

✦ **Physically,** you might experience aches and pains—tightness in your chest, a throbbing forehead—or sensations in your body from a past injury.

✦ **Behaviorally,** you could find yourself trying to hide, people pleasing, becoming argumentative.

BACKDRAFT IS PART OF THE HEALING PROCESS

Backdraft is a sign that self-compassion is working. It puts you in touch with those areas in yourself that need healing, including what you've been pushing out of awareness while going through burnout. If you're a burned-out physician, for example, and have a quiet moment to yourself, you might discover that you've started resenting your patients. Furthermore, you might feel shame for feeling resentment. None of this feels good, but it's good that it's coming up, because you can do something about it. You can treat yourself with compassion. Just notice what's arising—thoughts, emotions, sensations, behaviors—and treat yourself as you would treat a good friend. Even if you're not entirely sure what's going on inside you, be compassionate with yourself just *because* you feel bad. You'll probably find yourself becoming more compassionate again.

The most important thing to know about backdraft is that it's okay and you'll be okay. Actually, if you stick with the practice of self-compassion, you'll be *more* than okay.

When backdraft stirs up old wounds from the past, even from earliest childhood, you can update those childhood memories by responding to them in a new way—perhaps the way you wished you'd been treated many years ago. We're adults now, we know our needs better than others did in the past, and we have the resource of self-compassion to tend to our wounds. We can even *reparent* ourselves by responding compassionately to younger versions of ourselves, one memory at a time.

> **Backdraft feels like ka-boom, but it's really ka-*bloom!***

A WORD ABOUT SAFETY

We never know for sure what will arise as backdraft. It could be anything from a bit of uneasiness to major trauma. Self-compassion is powerful medicine, and as with all powerful medicines, we need to administer the right dose. As you practice self-compassion, please keep in mind the zones of tolerance that appear in the diagram on the next page.

The ideal balance for self-compassion practice is to feel challenged but to explore just a bit beyond your comfort zone. You don't want to be too safe, and you definitely don't want to be overwhelmed. When you feel entirely safe, you

Zones of Tolerance

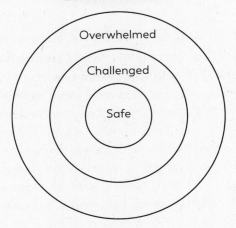

might not be motivated to learn. When you feel overwhelmed, you're causing yourself unnecessary stress and probably can't learn anything anyway.

Try asking yourself the following questions to determine what zone you're in:

- "How do I know when I feel **overwhelmed**?" Some signs are feeling flooded with emotion, self-doubt, tension, confusion, racing thoughts, distractedness, anger, dread, or exhaustion.

- "How do I know when I feel **challenged**?" Maybe you feel energized, curious, focused, alert, motivated, open-minded, or more creative.

- "How do I know when I feel **safe**?" Chances are you'll be feeling comfortable, content, friendly, grateful, or calm, your pulse will be slow and regular, and your breathing deep and steady.

Some people become captivated by the relief that self-compassion can bring. Then, if they feel overwhelmed by backdraft, they don't want to lower the dose of self-compassion. They imagine that more self-compassion will bring them relief. Unfortunately, that approach just brings more backdraft and more overwhelm. The solution to this dilemma is to practice self-compassion in a different way.

HOW TO WORK WITH BACKDRAFT

What should you do when backdraft arises? What you do depends on the zone of tolerance you're in. The rule of thumb is "lean in, lean back, or let go" of the practice. If you feel overwhelmed, move toward safety.

If backdraft comes up and you feel a bit anxious, but not much more, all you may need to do is remind yourself, "Oh, this is backdraft." Naming backdraft will give you a little distance from, or perspective on, what you're feeling. Then carry on with your self-compassion practice and see if the backdraft passes on its own.

When you feel *challenged* by backdraft, but not overwhelmed, you might wish to lean in and explore what's coming up for you. For example, if you're in the habit of keeping a journal, you could write down any memories that are arising, especially through a compassionate lens. You can also name the emotions that you're having—"sadness," "fear," "shame"—in a validating way, as you might for a friend. You can also explore where the emotion is felt most strongly in your body. (See Chapter 10 for more on this practice.) After doing all this, if you still feel uncomfortable, it might be time to back off a bit.

> When it comes to emotions, a good rule of thumb is "lean in, lean back, or let go."

If you ever feel *overwhelmed* by backdraft, the most self-compassionate thing to do is stop doing the practice. That doesn't mean that you have to stop practicing self-compassion altogether—you just need to practice self-compassion differently. When most people think about self-compassion practice, they think about *mental* training, like meditation. However, self-compassion practice is mostly *behavioral*—self-compassionate acts scattered throughout the day. You can't meditate all day long, so what you *do* in your life is the best indication of how self-compassionate you are.

If you find yourself struggling for any reason and take compassionate action on behalf of yourself, you're practicing self-compassion in daily life. Unfortunately, when we struggle, we often beat up on ourselves or hide in shame and are not kind to ourselves at all. Yet when we perform ordinary acts of self-care *as a response to suffering*—with behaviors like listening to music, gardening, or talking with friends—self-care becomes self-compassion. Behavioral self-compassion is what makes self-compassion safe for everybody. You just need to remember to do it!

To practice self-compassion in daily life, just ask yourself, "How do I usually care for myself?" You already have many good self-care habits, or you wouldn't have made it to adulthood. What are they? Some categories to consider are:

- **Physical.** Exercise, get a massage, take a warm bath, sip a cup of tea.
- **Mental.** Read an uplifting book, watch a funny movie, make some art.
- **Emotional.** Have a good cry, write in a journal, listen to music.
- **Relational.** Meet with friends, play with a pet, look at holiday photos.
- **Spiritual.** Pray, walk in the woods, help others.

If you like, you can make a list of activities that you enjoy and keep it as a handy reminder when you need some self-compassion.

There is also a practice you can do when you experience backdraft that can help you stand your ground, literally.

SELF-COMPASSION TOOL 7
Soles of the Feet

A proven way to move toward safety is to anchor your attention in the sensations of your feet. Your feet are as far from your head as possible, and the head is where most of our misery is manufactured. Focusing on your feet gets you out of your head and into your body, and feeling the *sensations* of your feet connects you with the earth. That feeling will be even more palpable if you're in a place where you can take off your shoes and literally feel the earth.

- ✦ If you can stand up, please do so. If you're unable to walk, you can adapt the following instructions and explore the sensations of your body being supported by your chair.
- ✦ Begin by noticing the sensations—the sense of touch—in the soles of your feet on the floor.
- ✦ To better feel sensation in the soles of your feet, try gently rocking forward and backward on your feet and side to side. Perhaps make little circles with your knees, feeling the changing sensations in the soles of your feet.

- Feel how the floor supports your whole body.
- When your mind has wandered, just begin feeling the soles of your feet again.
- Now begin walking, slowly, noticing the changing sensations in the soles of your feet. Notice the sensation of lifting a foot, stepping forward, and then placing the foot on the floor. Now do the same with the other foot. And then one foot after another.
- As you walk, perhaps appreciate how small the surface area of your feet is and how your feet support your entire body. If you wish, allow a moment of gratitude for the hard work that your feet are doing, which we usually take for granted.
- If you like, you can imagine an imprint of kindness or compassion on the floor with each step—whatever legacy you hope to leave behind in your life.
- Continue walking, slowly, feeling the soles of your feet.
- And then eventually return to standing again, expanding your awareness to your entire body, letting yourself feel whatever you're feeling and letting yourself be just as you are.

This practice tends to stop backdraft in its tracks. If backdraft continues, you can switch to some form of behavioral self-care like having a cup of tea.

You can also adapt the soles-of-the-feet practice to different work situations. Anxious about a hospital patient who's taken a downturn? Feel the soles of your feet as you walk toward or away from the patient's room. Urgently stopped by your boss while heading home after a long, hard day? Rock back and forth on your feet, and feel the changing sensations in your feet, as your boss explains the many things you still need to do but don't have time for.

Ben was a man continually on the move, so he liked it when Sybil suggested he try the soles-of-the-feet practice. It gave him a chance to calm his mind after work, especially when Sybil walked alongside him. Ben also enjoyed playing with his dog at the end of a long day. Both of these activities were acceptable self-compassion practices because they were expressions of self-care that didn't kick up any backdraft for Ben.

Self-compassion is a way of relating with kindness to any painful situation, including backdraft. A key part of the practice, therefore, involves being gentle and supportive toward yourself if compassion stirs up old pain. It's not shameful to admit that you're experiencing backdraft, or that you're burned out, or feeling any form of suffering for that matter—it opens the door to healing. Knowing you're experiencing backdraft *while* you're experiencing it requires *mindfulness*. The next chapter expands on the role of mindfulness in easing burnout.

8

PUTTING THINGS IN PERSPECTIVE

Mindful Awareness

When the exhaustion and frustration of burnout strike, we stop seeing things clearly. We may be so busy trying to survive that we lose touch with what we're feeling, not noticing how strained our resources are. One day we find we can't even get out of bed, and then we start analyzing what happened. Mindfulness, the foundation of self-compassion, can help us gain clarity and perspective.

With mindfulness we turn toward and become aware of our present-moment experience, even when it's painful. You may be saying to yourself, "I'm all too aware of how hard things are during my day, thank you very much." But are you? We often don't acknowledge discomfort when it's getting in the way of an important goal and ignore signals of overwhelm.

Maggie is a new therapist who specializes in treating adults with early childhood trauma. It's tough work, but she's committed to it. She admires her clients' will to survive and their resolve not to be held hostage by their past, which keeps her going.

How does Maggie cope with the tragic stories she hears day after day? She has the usual supports, such as a peer supervision group, and she tries to exercise regularly. But her main strategy is simply to avoid thinking about her work once she gets home. The stress of her work still affects her, though. She has lost her appetite, and she's not sleeping well.

Sometimes the issue isn't ignoring our pain, but rather getting carried away by it. We become completely lost in our negative thoughts and emotions, to the point that we have no perspective on them. We ruminate on how bad things are, and with each round of rumination things appear worse. We use obsessive thinking to try to solve our problems, but we're more likely to become tangled up in mental knots.

Maggie also succumbed to this pattern. When she couldn't successfully keep her head in the sand, her clients' stories would start flooding in. She would review everything they said, getting increasingly worked up. How could that have happened to an innocent child! She would also review everything she said in her sessions, wondering if she could have responded differently, if she was effectively using the techniques she had learned in her practicum. This soon spiraled into a storyline of being incompetent, that she was a fraud, that she would probably make her clients' lives worse, not better. Within a year Maggie was ready to quit her job. Luckily an older therapist from her peer supervision group suggested that she learn about mindfulness to help her cope with the difficult feelings she was experiencing.

Mindfulness disentangles us from painful thoughts and emotions by giving us a little distance from them. It's important to note that this is not the same thing as "sugarcoating" difficulty through positive thinking or denying our negative feelings. Mindfulness helps us become aware of our distress with balance and clarity so we aren't so overwhelmed by it.

> **With mindfulness, instead of ignoring our feelings or getting lost in them, we gain balance and perspective.**

DIRECT AWARENESS

Mindfulness provides clarity by allowing us to be directly aware of our experience rather than filtering it through the lens of thought. Thoughts are used to *represent* our experience. They create a mental image of what's happening so we can make sense of it. We project our thoughts into the past or future, facilitating planning. Thoughts often contain judgments that allow us to decide whether something is good or bad for us. But thoughts can't experience reality directly.

Think of a peach, for example. You might use thought to imagine what it looks like or tastes like, or to consider whether you like peaches or whether peaches are in season and available in the local market. But you can't eat the thought of a peach. Mindfulness experiences directly, allowing us to be aware of touching, seeing, smelling, tasting, and eating that peach.

We spend the vast majority of our time interacting with the world through thought: What is that? What does it mean? Is it good or bad? Where did it come from? Do I like it? Can I get more? What's going to happen to it? What can I do about it? Thought is incredibly useful, but we're so used to relying on it that we often don't notice the difference between *thoughts about* reality and reality itself. Mindfulness involves dropping beneath the chattering mind into direct awareness of what's happening, right now, using the five senses.

YOUR THOUGHTS CAN TRICK YOU!

Why is it important to differentiate thinking about reality from directly experiencing it through mindfulness? Because our thoughts are often wrong. For instance, you might have bought a beautiful peach imagining how delicious it was going to be, only to find out that it's bland and mealy. Our thoughts also tend to exaggerate things. If I'm having trouble making a deadline, I might create a storyline of being an inept worker who will never get things done, that I'll lose my job, then get evicted from my home. How long does it take to go from "trouble making deadlines" to "homeless"? Thoughts can move almost as fast as the speed of light.

Experiencing emotional discomfort directly with mindfulness, especially by becoming aware of the sensations it produces in the body, can be more helpful than thinking about it. Body sensations move much more slowly than thoughts, and we're unlikely to be mentally hijacked by body sensations. For instance, if we're experiencing insomnia, we can use mindfulness to feel the agitation in our chest, which is a kind of tension or tingling. These sensations are easier to bear than the thought "I'll never fall asleep!" We can also notice that the sensations of sleeplessness are constantly changing. Sleeplessness is a temporary state. Eventually it will pass and we'll fall asleep, especially when we stop thinking about not sleeping.

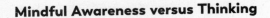

Mindful Awareness versus Thinking

Try exploring the difference between direct, mindful awareness and thinking:

✦ Start with **hearing.** Listen to the sounds coming at you in this moment. Just let them in and experience sound directly. Now let yourself *think* about the sounds. ("Oh, that's the air conditioner. Wow, that's loud. I wonder if I should get a quieter model.") Notice the difference between thinking about the sounds and hearing the sounds.

✦ Next gaze softly around you. **See** what's ahead, to your left, and to your right. Allow yourself to be aware of light, color, shapes, and so on, directly. Now engage your thinking. ("That's a lamp. One of its lightbulbs is out; I need to change it.") Notice the difference between thinking about what you see and just seeing.

✦ Pick up an object and **touch** it. Be aware of its texture, its softness or hardness. Run your hands over it. Now think about the object. ("That's a pen with green ink. I used it to sign my dinner check yesterday. Why would someone make a pen with green ink instead of blue or black?") Notice the difference between thinking about the object and feeling it.

✦ Next, take a sniff and see what you can **smell** in the air. Or raise your hand to your nose and smell your skin. Be aware of any scents you can detect. Now let yourself think about what you're smelling. ("My hands smell musty from the sponge I used to wash the dishes. Disgusting! I need to replace that sponge.") Notice the difference between thinking about the odor and just smelling it.

✦ Finally, notice any **tastes** in your mouth. Be directly aware of the experience of tasting. Then let your mind do what it naturally does—think. ("That's a poppy seed bagel I ate this morning. I also like blueberry bagels, but poppy seed is definitely my favorite.") Notice the difference between thinking about tastes and just tasting.

You can use mindfulness to become aware of the body sensations of burnout:

- Notice a feeling you're having right now related to burnout (such as exhaustion, stress, sadness, sleeplessness).

- Rather than thinking *about* the feeling or analyzing its causes, try dropping into your body and experiencing it directly.

- Where do you feel it in your body?

- Notice if the sensation is solid or vibrating.

- Is the sensation moving or changing?

- See if you can allow the sensation to be as it is, without ignoring, rejecting, or being carried away by thoughts about it.

The clarity that being mindful of our experience gives us is like standing still and looking into a clear pool of water with no ripples; it mirrors exactly what's happening—nothing added. Getting lost in our thoughts is more like looking at a video of waves rolling in, wondering how strong the undertow is, whether the water is freezing, and whether our swimming skills are up to the challenge.

Thoughts also fool us into thinking that our suffering will last forever. With mindful awareness we see that nothing is permanent. When we feel overwhelmed by all the tasks on our plate, our direct experience has nothing to say about how long those feelings will last. It's the thinking mind that makes predictions, so we not only feel overwhelmed but also fearful that we'll be overwhelmed forever. We worry we can't handle our stress and consider throwing in the towel.

That was certainly the corner Maggie had painted herself into, and she was eager for a way out. The colleague who introduced her to mindfulness recommended she try meditating to develop her mindfulness skills: in particular, to sit in silence and focus on her breathing. She said it would help Maggie calm and settle her mind. Maggie tried earnestly but quickly discovered that she could focus on her breath for only a few seconds before becoming distracted. Little did Maggie know that she had discovered the first insight of mindfulness meditation—the mind has a mind of its own. But why?

IT'S THE DEFAULT MODE NETWORK

Have you ever stepped out of the shower and found you couldn't remember if you had shampooed your hair, or pulled into your parking space with zero memory of driving to work? If so, you were probably in the thrall of the *default mode network*. This network of brain regions is one of our hardwired self-preservation systems. According to neuroscience, the default mode tends to be active when we're not paying attention to anything in particular (hence the term *default*). Unless we're intrigued by the task at hand, our minds have a natural tendency to wander and be consumed by thoughts. This is what happens when we meditate.

Where does the mind go? Well, mostly it goes in search of problems in the past and problems that could arise in the future ("I don't want *that* to happen to me again"). We also tend to think about our favorite subject—ourselves. When the brain is off duty for a little while, it becomes highly active planning how to keep us out of trouble. You can imagine how our worry-wart ancestors with an active default mode network were more likely to survive and pass their genes down than our chill forebears. Even when you're lying on a beach during a vacation, you're likely to be thinking about all the household chores and work tasks awaiting you back at home and start fretting about your ability to complete them. And you wonder why your last vacation didn't seem to ease your feelings of burnout?

Luckily, research shows that the more we practice mindfulness, the less we're trapped in the default mode. When we pay attention to our direct experience with our five senses, we unhook from the thinking mind and refocus on what's happening in the present moment. We give the mind something to do so it doesn't wander off into doom and gloom. What would happen if you tuned in to feeling exhausted or hopeless *without* the narration of your judgmental mind? These feelings would still be uncomfortable, but would they be as bad as you think? Yes, your situation is difficult. But what about this moment right now? Is it difficult? Are you safe? Are you alive? Can you find anything good about this moment that you overlooked? And if this moment is difficult, will it be difficult forever? Freeing our minds from the bondage of thought gives us the mental space to make choices about how to respond to the pain of burnout.

> **Mindful awareness frees up space in the mind for us to make new choices about how to respond to the distress of burnout.**

THE FIRST STEP TO SELF-COMPASSION

We need to be mindfully aware of our distress before we can give ourselves compassion. We can do this by intentionally asking ourselves, "What am I sensing? What am I feeling?" It's necessary to know that we're suffering before compassion makes any sense. If we block out our distress, or get caught up in the backstory and ruminate about it, we won't be in the frame of mind to ask, "What do I need right now that could help?" Maybe we need to take a break, or we need to get off the couch and take action. Could we use some words of comfort or encouragement? Maybe a reminder that we're not alone in this struggle?

Research has shown that the more you practice mindfulness, the more self-compassionate you become. When you can see through the BS story that your thoughts often create, you may realize that—at least in the moment—you're more okay than you thought. Mindfulness can help you remember that even if this moment is difficult, it will eventually pass. Mindfulness gives you a clear space to accept tough emotions—frustration, anger, resentment, despair—as normal human reactions to burnout.

Meditation is a classic way of learning and making a habit of mindfulness. Meditation is like going to the gym—it strengthens the mindfulness muscle, on purpose, for a dedicated period of time. But who has the energy to do mental training when stressed or burned out? Who wants to wrestle with their default mode network? And what if it just seems like another opportunity to "fail" at something? No worries; the following tool offers a way to meditate in a pleasant way, for just a few minutes, so you can disengage from the thoughts that cause unnecessary stress without worrying about getting it "right."

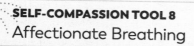

SELF-COMPASSION TOOL 8
Affectionate Breathing

You can do this practice anytime, even when taking a break in the middle of your workday. You don't need to strive for perfection, nor should this practice be a chore. A curious, almost playful, attitude is best. You can do it sitting in a chair, lying down, or standing up, whatever feels best and fits the situation you're in.

+ To start, please close your eyes, partially or fully, and drop your awareness inside your body. Take three deep breaths.

+ Scan your body to see if there are any places of stress, tension, or pain in your body, especially where you feel the *most* discomfort.

+ Then, if it feels right, put a hand on that place in your body. You can also put a hand over your heart or another soothing place. Simply feel the touch of your hand on your body.

+ Now begin to notice your breathing, feeling your body naturally breathe in and breathe out.

+ Start to notice the *rhythm* of your breathing, flowing in and flowing out. Take some time to *feel* the natural rhythm of your breathing.

+ Feel your *whole body* subtly moving with the breath, like the movement of the sea.

+ Allow your whole body to be gently rocked and caressed by your breathing.

+ Let yourself be aware that this gentle movement is always occurring in your body, no matter what you may be going through.

+ Feel the gentle rhythm for as long as you like. When your mind wanders, as it always will, just return to the rhythm of your breathing, giving yourself permission to savor the gentle flow.

+ And finally, release your attention to your breathing and allow yourself to feel whatever you're feeling and to be just as you are.

This type of breath meditation became Maggie's go-to practice when she wanted to relax. She particularly liked noticing the rhythm of her breathing, which made her feel like she was floating on a gentle ocean. When Maggie went to work in the morning, she took this practice with her. Her clients were scheduled with ten minutes between sessions, so in that precious time interval Maggie made it a habit to scan her body for areas of stress and then feel the rhythm of her breathing. She also allowed her body to gently sway back and forth with the rhythm of her breath. Five minutes was usually enough to let go of what had transpired in the previous session and get ready for her next client. When Maggie opened the door, she made sure she could feel the doorknob in her fingers. Then she smiled and welcomed her client.

Sometimes the thinking mind works against us: blaming ourselves for being burned out, creating unrealistic expectations, and catastrophizing about the future. Fortunately, with simple mindfulness skills we can free ourselves from unproductive thinking and respond more effectively to stress. But mindfulness isn't just about paying attention; it's also about *how* we pay attention: with acceptance instead of resistance. The next chapter explores how we can ease our feelings of burnout by letting go of unnecessary resistance.

9

RESISTANCE IS FUTILE

How Fighting Burnout Makes It Worse

Our first instinct when confronted with work stress is to ignore it or fight against it. Resistance is the struggle that occurs when we want our moment-to-moment experience to be other than it is. When we can't accept what's happening, we resist it. The term *resistance*, as we use it here, doesn't refer to engaging in social activism or fighting against the unjust systems that contribute to burnout. In fact, fighting for a more just future depends on accepting that injustice is occurring. Similarly, healing from burnout depends on accepting that burnout is occurring. When we resist the reality of burnout, it's harder to overcome it. Resistance causes our mind, heart, and body to contract, and that contraction exacerbates stress.

It's understandable that we resist the experience of chronic stress because it's so painful. The stress feels intolerable, and we want to make it go away immediately—yesterday in fact. So instead of accepting that this is how it is right now and working toward making things better in the future, we repress how we feel (which causes tension) or we get frustrated (which causes tension) or we blame ourselves (the icing on the tension cake).

Maria is an elementary school teacher in a small California town. She's extremely dedicated to her work and cares deeply about her students' right to a good education—many of them are children of undocumented immigrants who are struggling financially. On top of everything, after the recent spate of school shootings, she has been constantly worried about her students' safety. She has to conduct regular "active shooter" drills with her kids as they role-play what to do if it happens in their school. Maria must think about which students might not be able to follow directions due to special needs or language barriers or trauma—or which students she might have to pick up and carry.

Maria is upset by the way the administration conducts the active shooter drills, which terrify many of her students. She's also sickened by the horrifying reality that led the administration to implement the drills in the first place. Maria's feelings of frustration and despair follow her home at night and are utterly exhausting. She sometimes pounds her fists on her kitchen counter and screams, "This is not what teaching elementary school should be like!" Recently, she developed an ulcer and had to take two months' sick leave. Then she felt like a failure for letting her kids down.

RESISTING OUR EXPERIENCE

Resistance typically occurs in one of two ways, and you might be familiar with both of them: fighting and avoidance. Sometimes, like Maria, we *fight* against what is. We rail against reality and get angry and frustrated, as if somehow we can beat reality into submission. Think about times you've been caught in a traffic jam while running late for an important meeting. Honking your horn and strangling the steering wheel doesn't get you there any faster, but it certainly makes your drive more stressful. Fighting reality activates our sympathetic nervous system and makes us agitated. When we're already stressed and overwhelmed, wishing it were otherwise just makes us *more* stressed and overwhelmed.

Another, perhaps more subtle, form of resistance is trying to avoid our experience by denying what we're feeling. We dismiss our stress and ignore those feelings of exhaustion. "I don't have time to whine about a little backache," we mutter to ourselves, or "Other people have it worse than I do, so who am I to complain?" We reject our emotions as a sign of weakness and simply carry on. Some people avoid their emotions by zoning out to TV or drinking a little too much after work.

Although it would be nice if avoiding our difficulties made them go away, it doesn't work that way. We may ignore our stress or tiredness or our aching bones, but our bodies are affected regardless. We may distract ourselves from our feelings of overwhelm and hopelessness, but they're still there, simmering just below our conscious awareness. Research shows that suppressing unwanted thoughts and feelings just intensifies them when they inevitably pop up to the surface.

Whether it's through battling or ducking the problem, resistance rarely produces good solutions to our work stress. It doesn't make the pain go away; instead, it locks it in place. As the Borg aliens said in *Star Trek,* resistance is futile!

What we resist persists and grows stronger.

RESISTANCE IS NOT ONLY FUTILE—IT'S HARMFUL

Resisting our feelings of stress, overwhelm, and burnout is like slapping ourselves in the face. Even though we want to help ourselves by resisting pain, we end up harming ourselves instead. Sometimes suppressing emotional pain can be temporarily helpful and necessary. If you're a doctor who has to tell a young patient they have terminal cancer, you may need to compartmentalize—put some of your feelings in an imaginary drawer—so you can continue to function for the rest of the day. But over the long term, resistance takes a costly toll. If you never open that drawer and process the grief that you've been experiencing, it will come back to haunt you.

There's a simple equation to describe this phenomenon:

$$\text{Pain} \times \text{Resistance} = \text{Suffering}$$

In other words, we already feel the pain of work stress, but how much we suffer is directly related to how much we resist the pain in the first place. If we don't resist, it hurts. If we resist, not only does it hurt, but we also hurt ourselves through our resistance. The zombie feelings many burned-out people describe—feeling disconnected from their bodies and other people—are often a direct reflection of resistance to work stress. We shut down to avoid feeling pain and chronic stress, but how much fun is it to feel like a zombie?

We're surrounded by examples of how resisting our experience contributes to burnout:

- Suppressing your sadness over lack of support can contribute to depression.
- Fighting your fear of losing your job can lead to panic attacks.
- Ignoring your body's need for sleep can result in exhaustion.
- Railing against unavoidable work demands can raise your blood pressure.
- Pretending you're not overwhelmed will ensure that you remain overwhelmed.

HAVE YOU BEEN RESISTING THE PAIN OF WORK STRESS?

Sometimes we aren't aware that we're resisting the pain associated with work stress or burnout. Are you noticing any of the following signs of resistance in your life?

- ❑ Being spacy or distracted
- ❑ Getting lost in rumination or worry
- ❑ Feeling muscle aches and tension
- ❑ Overeating or drinking too much alcohol
- ❑ Feeling irritable
- ❑ Feeling empty or numb

COMPASSION RATHER THAN RESISTANCE

We mustn't judge ourselves for resisting pain. Even an amoeba will move away from a toxin in a petri dish. All biological organisms resist pain. It's normal and natural. But given how ineffective it is, we need to find a better way to cope with our stress. Instead of rejecting stress out of hand, we can give ourselves compassion because stress hurts.

As explored in the last chapter, self-compassion rests on the foundation of mindfulness. Mindful acceptance immediately ends our resistance as we let go of struggling with the reality of what is. It enables us to open to the truth of our experience without avoidance or rumination. But self-compassion involves more than mindfulness.

> Mindfulness asks, "What am I *experiencing* right now?"
> Self-compassion adds, "What do I *need* right now?"

These two questions allow us to take care of ourselves in the moment instead of veering off into rehashing the past, worrying about the future, and solving the "problem" of our own pain.

Tender self-compassion allows us to accept ourselves and our emotions with loving, connected presence when we feel burned out. We use mindfulness to be present with our stressful feelings, calling up the courage to turn toward them and be with them as they are. But we also use kindness to soothe and comfort ourselves because we're hurting, perhaps even putting a gentle hand on our body as a gesture of support. We remember that our feelings of burnout connect us to others. Burnout is everywhere in society, and we certainly aren't alone. There's also nothing wrong with us for feeling as we do—it's a sign of our humanity. When we hold the stress and frustration of our work with tender self-compassion, it becomes easier to bear.

THE PARADOX OF SELF-COMPASSION

The fact that mindful acceptance lies at the core of self-compassion creates what we like to call the central paradox of self-compassion: we give ourselves compassion not to feel better but *because* we feel bad.

You might find this confusing (it's a paradox, after all). You might also be a little peeved. *I thought I bought this book so I can feel better and not so burned out! I want my money back!* Of course we want to ease the symptoms of burnout and feel better. But improvement arises naturally from a new way of relating to our work stress. We can't throw self-compassion at our stress to extinguish it the way we might throw baking soda on a fire. If we try to use self-compassion as a slick new way of getting rid of what we're feeling in the moment, it's just resistance in another form. It won't work, because what we resist persists and grows stronger.

> **The paradox of self-compassion practice is that we give ourselves compassion not to feel better but because we feel bad.**

Maria discovered the importance of this paradox herself. A fellow teacher told her about the Self-Compassion for Educators course we created in conjunction with the Mindful Schools program. It's a six-week online program that provides self-compassion training for teachers. Participants get the highlights of the full MSC course and learn how to apply compassion in the midst of their workday. Maria took the course and found that self-compassion made a big difference in her ability to cope with the frustration and stress of her job. The practice that helped Maria the most was supportive touch (see Chapter 5). Maria grew up in a physically affectionate and loving Mexican American family. Her mother always gave her hugs and kisses when she was upset. The first time she gently put her hands on her heart in response to her distress she started to tear up. She heard her mother's voice say, "It's okay, Chiquita. I'm here for you." She was surprised by how the tension eased and was easier to endure. She started to put her hands on her heart whenever she was stressed, even in the classroom. She wasn't embarrassed about it. She told everyone she could about the power of self-compassion.

But after a while Maria noticed that self-compassion wasn't working anymore. After a tense meeting with her principal to discuss the active shooter drills, for instance, Maria put her hands on her heart, but nothing happened—she remained as upset as ever. Was she doing it wrong? Then she remembered learning about the central paradox in the self-compassion course. Her intention had shifted subtly. Instead of putting her hands on her heart to comfort and soothe herself because she felt bad, Maria was putting her hands on her heart to feel better—to make her bad feelings go away.

As soon as Maria realized this, she tried again. She accepted and acknowledged how tense she felt and put her hands on her heart as a simple sign of warmth and care. As she stopped contracting in reaction to her distress, the tension started to ease. *Why* Maria put her hand on her heart—the subtle motivation behind the act—made all the difference.

Cultivating acceptance doesn't contradict taking action to improve the conditions of our workplace. Fierce self-compassion is all about speaking up and making change (more on fierce self-compassion in the chapters ahead). But the motivational force of fierce self-compassion is aimed at the future. We can't make needed changes if we avoid our problems right now or don't accept what we're feeling. And if we're so frustrated by fighting the reality of our situation that we lose perspective, how are we going to take effective action or make a meaningful difference? Tender and fierce self-compassion are both necessary to reduce the suffering caused by burnout.

Because resistance to work-related stress can be counterproductive, it's helpful to start noticing how you're unconsciously resisting and consider how self-compassion may shift things. The following exercise is designed to help you do this.

SELF-COMPASSION TOOL 9
Reducing Resistance to Work-Related Stress

Please reflect on the following questions (and write your answers if you like):

✦ Bring to mind what causes stress in your work. For example, it might be your workload, the type of work you do, difficult people, inadequate pay, too many hours, unsafe conditions, challenging clients, or job insecurity. Then choose the *most* stressful aspect of your work.

✦ How are you relating to the stress caused by this aspect of your work? For example, if your customers are angry or disrespectful, how do you cope? Are you avoiding or denying your stress (perhaps procrastinating on a work deadline or zoning out on TV after a long day caring for Mom)? Are you fighting or railing against it (maybe complaining loudly to others or getting irritated a lot)?

✦ Think of the short-term benefits that your resistance may be offering you (such as reducing the intensity of your emotions or giving you a feeling of control).

✦ Consider the long-term costs of your resistance. Might it be causing you more stress and making your burnout worse over time (like creating even more pressure to complete work or damaging your relationships with coworkers)?

✦ Consider what could happen if you tried to accept the present-moment reality of your stress instead of resisting it. How might things change for you?

- See if you can provide some tender self-compassion for the stress you're experiencing right now. For example, can you use supportive touch combined with some words of kindness, comfort, or care to acknowledge the stress you feel? Does this shift anything for you?

- Also consider how fierce self-compassion (taking action) might help you reduce your stress in the future (perhaps by speaking to your supervisor, taking time for yourself, drawing boundaries, or doing things differently). Are there any small changes you could make that might help?

After doing this exercise, Maria could see how her resistance to her stress wasn't helping. Fuming to herself all day about the school administration's policies just made her more stressed, and nothing changed. When she brought in self-compassion, however, things became a bit easier. Acknowledging her frustration and fear and extending real warmth and compassion for the difficult situation she and her students were in—especially after all the terrifying school shootings—softened something inside her. She felt less contracted, almost as if there was more space in her body to hold all the tension.

Fierce self-compassion was also important for Maria. Part of her resistance came from wanting to change things for the better. So she decided that she was going to try to alter the way her school held the active shooter drills so they were less frightening to students. She started reading everything she could on the subject, talked to other teachers, and gathered options for the administration. She didn't know if her efforts would make a difference, but she was going to try.

It's understandable to resist pain and stress and to want to make it go away—who doesn't? But unfortunately, banging our head again the wall of reality just gives us a headache. Once we lessen our resistance with mindfulness and self-compassion, we have more resources available to take action to change our stressed-out, burned-out world.

Granted, it's easier said than done to simply drop your resistance to pain and stress. There's a reason we resist our difficult emotions—they can feel like a hurricane blowing us away, causing us to lose our footing and our bearings. There are specific mindfulness and compassion techniques that can help you work more skillfully with difficult emotions when they arise, which we explore in the next chapter.

10

FACING THE STORM

Working with the Difficult Emotions of Burnout

Burnout involves a boatload of difficult emotions. First there are the feelings of stress, frustration, and exhaustion that drive burnout. Then there are the emotional companions of burnout: hopelessness, cynicism, dejection, grief, anger, resentment, anxiety. Finally, there are the ways we feel about ourselves for being burned out—shame, blame, and disappointment. We can easily be overwhelmed by all these painful emotions.

Burnout is a kind of coping mechanism that we unconsciously adopt to deal with our chronic distress. We shut down, go numb, develop brain fog, and become detached, because remaining open and vulnerable to our pain feels unbearable. Of course, no one chooses burnout as an intentional coping strategy, but the mind and body close as naturally as an armadillo that rolls up into its shell when attacked by a dog. Burnout can be seen as a method of self-preservation. When we can't get out of bed, we aren't working so hard. When we're numb, we don't hurt as much. When we can't think straight, we don't have to constantly focus on our problems. When we're cynical, our hopes can't be dashed so easily. When we believe we're utter failures, we can't sink any lower.

Klara is a psychiatrist in a large clinic who worked to get her medical degree and psychiatry specialization because she wanted to help people. But she has so many patients that she can spend only a few minutes with each one, and she devotes most of her time to paperwork. Even when Klara is with a patient, she's mainly entering information into her notes. She went into the profession to do hands-on work that could make a real difference to people with mental illness, but her main clients these days seem to be the insurance companies.

At first this deeply troubled Klara, but lately she doesn't feel much of anything. She goes through the motions of her job like an automaton, even though she tries to smile and hide her apathy. There's something slightly protective about being in that detached state. It numbs the pain of watching her dream of helping people evaporate. Klara worries about how cynical she's become, however. She finds herself using belittling nicknames for her patients, like "endless talker," "drama queen," and "walking disaster." She's starting to question her empathy skills and her decision to specialize in psychiatry. Blaming herself is also a distraction from feeling she has no power over the broken mental health care system at the root of it all. Although Klara is shielding herself by shutting down, she's also shutting out the possibility of improving her work or her life.

Dealing with emotional pain by numbing it, distracting ourselves, or becoming resigned cynics is only a temporary fix. We can't avoid pain forever. As noted in the last chapter, what we resist persists and grows stronger. But being at the end of our rope in a state of burnout can also be a gift, because it highlights the fact that we've run out of escape routes. The only way out is *through*. Eventually we need to turn toward our pain and look it straight in the face. To do this we need to wrap ourselves in the protective cloak of self-compassion, which helps us make this turn slowly and safely.

APPROACHING DIFFICULT EMOTIONS WITH A STRONG BACK AND SOFT FRONT

Often our reactions to the imperfection of life, including chronic work stress and our limited capacity as humans to deal with it, are driven by fear. Joan Halifax, a Buddhist meditation teacher and writer, says that when fear is powering our reactions, we typically adopt a hard front (the critical cynic) to hide a weak back (lack of confidence that we can survive). She proposes that we turn this around when things get difficult, aiming instead to cultivate a strong back but a soft front. Having a strong back means we're courageous and firm but also flexible (trees that fail to bend with the wind snap, and so do humans). This strength provides the safety needed to open to our pain rather than defend ourselves from it. Having a soft front means we use compassion to comfort and care for ourselves because we hurt.

Facing chronic stress with compassion allows us to stand our ground as the winds swirl around us while keeping our hearts open. An incredible example of someone with a soft front and strong back was Rosa Parks, a Black woman living in the 1950s in racially segregated Montgomery, Alabama. She was asked to give up her seat in the "colored" section of the bus to a White passenger because the "White" section was filled. Politely and respectfully, she refused. She was tired of her people being mistreated, so she sat with her head held high and didn't budge. Her profound act of courage and compassion helped to spark the civil rights movement and end legal segregation in the United States.

We can adopt a similar stance toward the unrelenting emotional assault of our work lives. Instead of letting it eject us from our seat, we can decide not to budge and to face it head on. If we can hold ourselves with strength and love as we let ourselves *feel* what we're feeling, we don't become so overwhelmed. It's not dissimilar to holding a tantrumming two-year-old with firmness and tenderness at the same time, letting them know we love them and that they have our support as they cry it out. Eventually the child will start to calm down. We can use the same approach to the emotions related to burnout.

But Klara hadn't learned about self-compassion yet, unfortunately, and her back wasn't strong. One day she walked into her office and found papers all over the floor next to her desk. Apparently, the pile of patient files had gotten precariously high and toppled over, with loose papers cascading to the ground. She went limp and considered dumping them all in the wastebasket. What did it matter anyway?

Then she glanced at a paper in her hand and recognized the name of a brave transgender teen who struggled with depression after being bullied and rejected at school, who just wanted to be accepted for who he was. He mattered. A crack appeared in Klara's armor. The pain and frustration and anger and feelings of despair started to pour in, and they kept coming until finally she collapsed on the floor alongside the papers. She was knocked flat. The doors of Klara's heart opened too suddenly, and she didn't have a solid self-compassion practice to stand on, so she was swept away by the flood of her repressed feelings.

TAKING IT GRADUALLY

Difficult emotions can be overwhelming if we open to them too quickly. It's important to take it gradually, making sure we have the strength and resources needed to cope moment by moment. We have a saying in the self-compassion world: "Walk slowly, go farther." In other words, we set our intention to open to our pain and let go of resistance, but do it little by little, so that we can build up strength along the way. The process of letting go of resistance to our emotions typically goes through five stages, known as the *stages of acceptance* (shown in the box).

When dealing with chronic stress, our usual way of relating to it is with resistance. We ignore it or are taken over by it, fueling burnout. The first step toward acceptance is simply to identify what you're feeling. You recognize that you're stressed. The next step involves feeling the stress in your body, perhaps as tension in your neck and shoulders. Tolerating means you're making more direct

The Five Stages of Acceptance

1. **Resisting:** This is where most of us start. We desperately want the painful emotions to go away, so we either pretend they aren't there or fight against them. Unfortunately, neither strategy works.

2. **Exploring:** We peep through the keyhole to see who's there. Turning toward our difficult emotions with curiosity, we ask, "What am I feeling?" We do this more cognitively than emotionally, however.

3. **Tolerating:** Once some stability has been established, we tolerate the reality of our painful emotions. We feel them but still wish they would go away.

4. **Allowing:** At the next step we give up our resistance and allow the painful feelings in. We fully accept our emotional experience as it is.

5. **Befriending:** Finally, we start to see value in our difficult emotions, realizing that they often have an important gift of growth or learning for us.

contact with the feeling, even though you still want the stress to go away. In the phase of allowing, you give up the agenda for the stress to go away. You accept that you're stressed and make space for it in your awareness. Finally, you start to realize that the feeling of stress is giving you an important message. Instead of resenting feeling stressed, you're grateful that it's pointing out that you're overworked and need to slow down. Once we befriend our difficult emotions, they're no longer so difficult. By changing our relationship to our pain, we help ourselves suffer less.

Feeling grateful for difficult emotions can be a tall order, however, which is why it's important to go slowly and only at a pace that feels safe. You can always back off for a little while if needed. For instance, becoming overloaded with adrenaline after trying to tolerate the feelings of stress in your body would be a clear sign to disengage and go back to simply mentally noticing that the stress is there. You want to move forward only once that feels safe (perhaps after taking a walk or talking to a friend). Working with difficult emotions requires self-compassion.

Walk slowly, go farther.

STRATEGIES FOR OPENING TO DIFFICULT EMOTIONS RELATED TO BURNOUT

Difficult emotions are temporary. Left to their own devices, they arise, are felt for a while, then pass on. When we resist our feelings, however, we lock them into place so they can't naturally fade away. That's why it's so important to try to let go of resistance when it feels safe to do so. To let go of resistance to challenging feelings and work toward accepting them, consider the following three techniques rooted in mindfulness and compassion.

Labeling emotions: You can explore a difficult emotion that arises by giving it a name or label (fear, disappointment, stress, shame, and so forth). Gently repeat the name for the feeling when it comes up, noting what's there in an objective manner. When you name an emotion, you stop avoiding it, but you also keep yourself from getting lost in it. In effect, when you name what you're feeling you get some distance from it and are no longer caught by it. Labeling practice is an effective mindfulness tool for working with difficult emotions, and research has shown that using this strategy weakens the brain's tendency to become reactive and lessens activity in the amygdala.

Feeling emotions in the body: A useful mindfulness technique that can help you tolerate difficult emotions is to *feel* the emotion as a physical sensation in your body. All emotions have a mental and physical component. The emotion of fear, for example, may be driven by the thought "I'm way behind and I'll lose my job," but also express itself physically as churning in the stomach. We're such thought-based creatures that we tend to focus mainly on what's happening, why it shouldn't be happening, and who's to blame for it. Focusing instead on the physical experience of our emotions helps us disentangle from our thoughts, where our resistance lies.

Soften–soothe–allow: A compassion-based process we call *soften–soothe–allow* can help you learn to make space for difficult emotions and even befriend them. While experiencing an emotion as a physical sensation, you orient toward it with softness and tenderness, relaxing the constriction in the body. You then soothe,

- **Softening—physical compassion**
- **Soothing—emotional compassion**
- **Allowing—mental compassion**

comfort, and support yourself *because* you're hurting and in emotional pain. Finally, with the strength and safety offered by your own care, you simply allow your experience to be as it is. Because resistance increases suffering, letting go of resistance is an act of self-compassion.

You can use the two mindfulness techniques of labeling difficult emotions and feeling them in your body as stand-alone practices. Adding compassion to the mix is especially powerful, however. A really good time to use the following tool, which combines all three approaches, is when you're in bed at night and your mind is racing with distressing thoughts and feelings.

SELF-COMPASSION TOOL 10
Being with Difficult Emotions Related to Burnout

Become aware of a situation related to your experience of burnout that's generating difficult emotions—having too much work to do, getting too little sleep, dealing with a broken administrative system, and so on. Play out the situation in your mind's eye—what's happening and who is involved, if anyone.

- **Label** any difficult emotions that are arising, such as stress, disappointment, grief, fear, hopelessness, shame, inadequacy, and confusion. You may also notice and label a lack of emotion (such as numbness). See if you can identify the strongest emotion you're experiencing and repeat the label for that emotion in a friendly way.

- **Drop out of your head and into your body.** Focusing on the emotion you've named, see if you can identify where you actually *feel* the emotion as a physical sensation. Pounding in your head, constriction in your throat, twisting in your gut, or another sensation? If you can't identify a specific place in your body where the emotion resides, see if you can sense any physical tension or discomfort. As much as possible, let go of the storyline driving the emotion and simply feel your body.

- **Soften** your body around the physical sensation of the emotion without trying to change it. Hold it a bit more tenderly, relaxing around the edges, allowing the tension to melt slightly.

- **Soothe,** comfort, and support yourself because it's hard to feel this emotion. You might place a warm hand on the place in your body where you feel the emotion or on some other comforting place. Silently speak some words of kindness and support, as you might use with a close friend: "I'm so sorry your situation is so difficult" or "I'm here for you."

- **Allow** your discomfort to be there. Create some space for it, letting go of any need to change it or make it go away, at least in this moment.

- If you like, stick with the emotion as a physical sensation, repeating "*soften–soothe–allow.*" You might find that other emotions arise or the location of the emotion shifts. Simply allow the emotions to do their dance, held in the safety of your own care and support.

When Klara learned this practice it made a big difference for her. She did it every night when she got into bed, asking herself what difficult emotions were triggered by her work that day. Typically they were feelings of frustration over the amount of paperwork she had. She would name the frustration and drop into her body to feel the tension in her chest. Then she would soften around the edges of the frustration. It was almost like she was perforating the edges of it so it wasn't so tightly bound. Then she put her hands on her chest, over her heart, and comforted herself for the pain she was experiencing. Using a warm and caring yet firm tone of voice, she would silently say things like "Of course you're upset, Klara. You want to help these people who are struggling with their mental health, but your hands are tied by all the paperwork. Anyone would feel frustrated. You're doing your best in difficult circumstances." She felt her own strength and the commitment to be there for herself. This support allowed her to let go of her resistance to the frustration and simply allow it to be there as a physical sensation. She imagined that the sensation was arising in a vast warm and loving space and that she actually was this vast and loving space. How can space be harmed?

Often when Klara did additional rounds of soften–soothe–allow, she would discover other emotions lying underneath the frustration—fear, anger, despair, grief. She would resolutely stick with whatever emotions came up, not budging, holding them with space and love. Eventually she began to experience a warm, peaceful feeling, and the difficult emotions would subside somewhat. Klara came to rely on this nightly practice to process and digest the emotional pain of her work so that she was no longer overwhelmed by it.

She also realized that her frustration had an important message for her: she needed to try to do something about the broken system. She joined a group of doctors who were advocating for insurance reform. Although it was an uphill battle, at least she was reengaged with the value of helping others that had led her to enter the mental health profession in the first place.

When we use a soft front and strong back to stay with the discomfort of difficult emotions, they tend to arise, do their little dance, then move on. We don't have to be knocked down by them. We don't have to shut down in a zombie-like state of burnout to avoid feeling them. By changing the way we relate to difficult emotions, we can get through almost any storm and live to fight another day.

Self-compassion not only helps us cope with our own difficult emotions, it also helps us cope with the difficult emotions of others, especially in caregiving situations. The next chapter examines how self-compassion can protect us from empathic distress, a common cause of burnout.

STOPPING THE DRAIN

Reducing Empathy Fatigue

For those who care for others on a daily basis, a key factor in creating burnout is the stress that stems from being around people in pain, also known as *empathic distress*. This will be no surprise to first responders, health care professionals, family caregivers, clergy members, or social activists, who are often depleted by their continual exposure to others' suffering. Sensitivity to distress and the desire to alleviate suffering often draw caregivers to their work in the first place, but the more you care, the more vulnerable you are to burnout.

When you're deeply invested in helping those in need, you tend to give it all you've got, even when your personal resources are draining away. You selflessly work long hours, even past the point of exhaustion, when you're called to do so. Self-compassion is needed to stop the drain. Without offering yourself support, kindness, and comfort, you can't expect to go on like this forever.

But it's not just overwork driven by dedication and perseverance that causes the drain. It's feeling the distress of others as if it's your own.

"I FEEL WHAT YOU FEEL"

Empathy is the capacity of the human brain to resonate with the emotions of others at a preverbal level. When others feel sad, we feel sad. When others laugh, we laugh. When others are tense, we feel tense. This ability evolved to secure our own survival and that of the species. Parents who could feel what their infants were feeling before they learned to speak were more likely to meet their needs effectively, so their children lived to pass on their genes to future generations. The ability of group members to resonate with one another's emotions, be it fear, anger, happiness, or contentment, was crucial for our hunter-gatherer ancestors to coordinate their interactions so the tribe could survive and thrive.

Our capacity for empathy is innate and natural. Recent years have seen significant research into the phenomenon of empathic resonance, with some suggesting that we have a particular type of neuron, called *mirror neurons,* designed specifically to relay information about what others are feeling. We know that human brains synchronize to share emotions. Research in a field sometimes referred to as *interpersonal neurobiology* shows that synchronization occurs between two people in everything from areas of brain activity to heart and breathing rates to pupil size and body movements.

Empathy often flows most easily with those we care about—family, friends, and loved ones—because we interact with them frequently and are more aware of their experience. But empathy for those who are suffering doesn't necessarily involve caring about their suffering. For instance, con artists can use empathy to sense when a mark is feeling confident or trusting and take advantage of their intended victim.

Empathy is generally beneficial and promotes social cohesion and interpersonal closeness, but it also has costs. When we're in the presence of those feeling physical pain or negative emotions such as fear, stress, sadness, or anger, we feel their pain directly. When we see a person accidentally slam a door on their finger, we flinch not only on behalf of that person, but because the pain centers in our own brains have been activated. For family caregivers who feel the distress of their loved one day after day, or for professional caregivers who deal with client after client in pain, empathy makes the job of caregiving even more stressful and draining. An ob-gyn witnessing a patient's grief over losing her unborn child also feels grief. A man caring for his depressed brother is likely to also feel depressed over time. The executive assistant whose boss is stressed and anxious feels their own breath quicken and heart race along with their employer's. It's hard enough feeling our own distress and frustration in the work we do, but as if we're in a multi-vehicle crash, we also feel everyone else's distress!

For twenty years, Martin has been the rector of an Episcopal church, where he has built an inclusive, welcoming environment for all who worship there. Over the years the church has become an important safe haven for many unhoused people in his parish, who come to the church for food or medical supplies and to Martin for comfort and advice. Martin seems tireless and sometimes must be coaxed back to the rectory late in the evening by his wife, Sheila. Sheila is worried about Martin. He's pale and seems distracted, and she knows that he often lies awake at night worrying about those souls in dire straits who are seeking aid or counsel.

Sheila sees on Martin's face the same pain etched into the faces of those standing in line for the Tuesday food pantry. She watches him walk with the same stoop as those who have lost hope of finding a job and come to him in despair to ask for his help. But when Sheila suggests they take a week's vacation and leave the church in the capable hands of the associate pastor, Martin straightens up, puts a smile on his face, and says he's fine.

Yet he's not fine. He's completely worn out and has recently started to sit staring into space in his study in the afternoon. His immune system is weakened, and he seems to catch every virus that's going around. Martin is an empathic guy who feels whatever his parishioners are feeling to the point where it's draining his own strength and resilience.

Secondary Traumatic Stress

When we empathize with those experiencing pain, we're at risk of suffering secondary traumatic stress. The term was coined when researchers noticed that first responders who dealt with traumas like car accidents or gunshot wounds were developing PTSD symptoms such as intrusive thoughts and memories, sweating, nausea, and trembling. Even though they weren't experiencing the trauma themselves, their minds and bodies were traumatized empathically, hence the term *secondary* traumatic stress. You don't have to witness actual blood and guts to be traumatized empathically. Anyone exposed to a high level of emotional, psychological, or physical pain—therapists, social workers, family caregivers, teachers—can be affected.

COMPASSION VERSUS EMPATHY

Some people use the term *compassion fatigue* as a synonym for secondary traumatic distress, or as a way to describe the emotional exhaustion and burnout

Are You Suffering from Secondary Traumatic Stress?

The U.S. Department of Health and Human Services describes secondary traumatic stress as involving a variety of cognitive, emotional, behavioral, and physical symptoms. If you regularly interact with people in physical or emotional pain, are you experiencing any of the following?

- ☐ Difficulty concentrating
- ☐ Difficulty breathing
- ☐ Elevated heart rate
- ☐ Hypervigilance
- ☐ Nightmares
- ☐ Persistent anger

- ☐ Difficulty sleeping
- ☐ Appetite changes
- ☐ Frequent illnesses
- ☐ Desire to avoid people
- ☐ Numbness
- ☐ Persistent sadness

experienced by caregivers. But compassion is not fatiguing. When we experience compassion, we feel others' pain, but we also feel care and concern. Compassion generates feelings of warmth and connection that are energizing and provide a buffer against the negative effects of empathic pain. In a research study that trained people in either compassion or empathy, scientists found that watching a movie that depicted suffering activated different networks in the brains of the two groups of participants. Empathy training activated the amygdala and was linked to negative feelings such as sadness, stress, and fear, while compassion training activated the reward centers of the brain and generated positive emotions like kindness and interest.

Caregivers experience empathy fatigue, not compassion fatigue.

When we feel compassion toward others who are suffering, we're less overwhelmed by their pain. First, kindness is a positive, fulfilling emotion that can replenish us and provide resources to cope. Our recognition of common humanity helps us feel connected to those in pain, while still understanding how self and other are distinct. And the element of mindfulness that is central to compassion keeps us from becoming fused or overidentified with negative emotions, as can occur with empathy.

One nurse who took our Self-Compassion for Healthcare Communities (SCHC) course reported, "I'm really good at connecting with people, and that's a good thing. But it also makes me really tired, and I'm vulnerable to getting really overloaded. I shouldn't have to have an emotional hangover for two days and be exhausted and want to hide at my house because I can't take any more on. For a long time I couldn't separate or didn't even know that I should be trying to separate someone else's emotion from mine, because to me they end up being the same thing sometimes. Self-compassion training helped me understand what I had read before—that there is a difference between compassion and empathy. Just because I'm feeling their pain doesn't mean it's mine."

Importantly, to counter the draining effects of empathy fatigue, compassion needs to be directed both outward and inward. We need to relate to our own empathic distress with caring, warmth, and strength while caring for others.

PUTTING ON YOUR OWN OXYGEN MASK FIRST

On every airline flight we're told that we need to put on our own oxygen mask before helping others. This metaphor is widely used for explaining why caregivers need to practice self-care to counter burnout. Typically people are referring to physical self-care such as yoga, massages, and sleep. Although self-care activities are important (see "Self-Care and Self-Compassion" in Chapter 16), they are of little help in the actual moment when our mirror neurons are buzzing with someone else's pain. We can't say, "Uh, excuse me, your sobbing is really freaking me out. I'm going to go get a massage!" However, while we're experiencing empathic pain, we can direct compassion toward ourselves.

As you're feeling the stress or intensity of another's pain, you can mindfully acknowledge your empathic distress: "This is so hard. I feel sad and confused and overwhelmed." You can realize that caring for others is a challenging but rewarding aspect of the human experience: "I'm not alone; all caregivers feel this way sometimes." And you can support yourself with the type of warm words you might naturally use with a friend: "I'm sorry you're having such a hard time. I'm here for you." Holding your empathic pain with compassion as you care for others provides a sense of calm, stability, and resilience.

And there's a bonus for doing so. Empathic resonance goes both ways. Just as we're impacted by the emotions of those we care for, other people are equally affected by our own internal mind states. When we're self-critical or irritated, others sense this through their mirror neurons and become more agitated. But when we're self-compassionate and our hearts are filled with loving, connected presence, others feel that presence. You might say that people can experience secondary self-compassion just like they experience secondary traumatic stress. When we turn our focus inward and give ourselves compassion for feeling the pain of others, they benefit from our open heart through empathic resonance. Our inner warmth lifts everyone up.

It's tragic that some family and professional caregivers don't practice self-compassion in the mistaken belief that it's selfish or self-centered. It's anything but.

Self-compassion is the most precious gift we can give to those we care for.

SELF-COMPASSION AND EQUANIMITY

Another way that self-compassion helps reduce empathy fatigue is by cultivating equanimity. When we criticize ourselves as caregivers, there's often an implicit agenda of control. We want to alleviate or eliminate the other person's suffering and feel we *should* be able to do so. Not only do we take on the emotions of others, but we also take on responsibility for their well-being. The wisdom of self-compassion reminds us that we have human limitations, and although we can try our best, we don't have power over the mental, psychological, or physical health of others. Self-compassion allows us to be humble and give up the illusion of control.

There are some equanimity phrases we teach in the SCHC program to help caregivers remember this truth, especially when they're working with a patient who is suffering:

Everyone is on their own life journey.

I am not the cause of this person's suffering,
nor is it entirely within my power to make it go away,
even though I wish I could.

Moments like this are difficult to bear,
yet I may still try to help if I can.

For many caregivers the wisdom of equanimity is the missing puzzle piece that allows them to open their heart to self-compassion. When we let go of expectations of omnipotence, we can rest more easily. Equanimity can be especially tricky for parents, but they eventually understand that even their own children have separate, unique experiences and life trajectories.

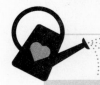

SELF-COMPASSION TOOL 11
Compassion with Equanimity

To practice self-compassion in the middle of a caregiving interaction, you can use this tool as a way of putting on your oxygen mask. In fact, it uses the breath as a metaphorical vehicle for compassion directed both inward and outward. It also uses the equanimity phrases provided on page 99, which can be memorized and spoken silently. This tool is designed to be used when you feel distressed while caring for someone in pain, but you may want to learn it first while imagining a caregiving situation *before* doing it in real time.

✦ Try giving yourself some sort of soothing and supportive touch. If you're in front of the person you're caring for, you may want to use a non-obvious touch like stroking your forearms or holding your own hand.

✦ Repeat these phrases silently to yourself, as a reminder to cultivate equanimity:

Everyone is on their own life journey.

I am not the cause of this person's suffering,
nor is it entirely within my power to make it go away,
even though I wish I could.

Moments like this are difficult to bear,
yet I may still try to help if I can.

✦ Feel the stress you are carrying in your body and breathe in deeply, drawing compassion inside your body and filling every cell of your body with compassion. Let yourself be soothed by inhaling deeply and giving yourself the compassion you need.

+ As you exhale, send out compassion to the person who is the source of your empathic pain. Imagine that every cell of their body is being filled with compassion.

+ Continue breathing compassion in and out, allowing your body to gradually find a natural breathing rhythm. "In for me, out for you." "One for me, one for you."

+ If you find that you need to focus primarily on giving compassion to yourself, give yourself full permission to do so. You can concentrate on your inbreath and only occasionally focus on your outbreath. "Six for me, one for you."

+ Imagine that there is an unlimited supply of compassion available in the air you are breathing, more than enough for you and the person you're caring for.

+ If you find yourself getting caught by the other's pain, try repeating the equanimity phrases.

+ Let go of the practice once you've found some equilibrium and don't feel overwhelmed by empathic pain.

Martin didn't find it easy to shift into self-compassion. He had learned in seminary that selflessness and self-sacrifice were the primary virtues of a pastor. He squirmed at giving himself kindness when so many in his flock were in such need. But one of his congregants was a doctor who had taken the SCHC program and taught him the compassion with equanimity tool. He began to use it at the Tuesday food pantry, putting his own spin on it. As he saw the depression and despair on the faces of many who took food boxes, he breathed out for them, sending them God's love. That wasn't new for him. What was new was getting in touch with his empathic pain—realizing how much his own heart was breaking. So he also sent himself God's love. He silently whispered words inspired by David's in Psalm 23:6: "May goodness and love follow me all of the days of my life." He allowed these words, along with the image of breathing compassion into every cell of his body, to comfort and soothe him.

But the equanimity phrases were what really shifted things for Martin, since they reminded him of the Serenity Prayer: "God, grant me the serenity to accept the things I cannot change, the courage to change the things I can, and the wisdom to know the difference." He realized that at some point he had felt like a good pastor should be able to alleviate the suffering of his congregation. When he got more perspective through the self-compassion practice, he recognized that, although his efforts were important and necessary, ultimately the lives of his flock were in more capable hands than his own. As he began to take the pressure off himself, he noticed that his strength gradually returned. He found he had more energy to give to others when his compassion flowed inward as well as outward.

We don't choose to experience empathic pain; it's part of our neurobiology. Luckily, we can counter its negative effects with self-compassion. But it does take some intentional effort to recognize how empathy fatigue is exacerbating our feelings of burnout and to turn compassion toward our empathic pain. Letting go of the illusion of control is also a game changer, especially for those with the personality trait of perfectionism.

Like empathy, perfectionism has costs as well as benefits. In the next chapter we explore the downsides of buying into society's message that we must be perfect to be worthy. Perfectionism may help us achieve our goals, but it can also derail us, especially when it results in burnout. Fortunately, self-compassion can help us let go of the need to always get it right.

WHEN GOOD ISN'T GOOD ENOUGH

Avoiding the Perfectionism Sinkhole

Caring about the work we do and trying to do our best at it are wonderful qualities, but they can have a dark side. When we judge our worth by our productivity and expect ourselves to be perfect, being a flawed human becomes a problem. Human beings (by definition) are imperfect, so perfectionism (by definition) is unachievable. Perfectionism says we're never doing enough, never good enough, and eventually we start to believe those messages. If it's not okay to fail, make mistakes, or achieve less than we're aiming for, we will never be at rest.

Kebede is a lawyer in New York who specializes in helping recent immigrants. His own family emigrated from Ethiopia when he was seven, and Kebede's father impressed on him the importance of excelling at school to succeed in their new country. Kebede developed into a perfectionist who always had to get things right. In school if he got an A– on an exam, he would get upset and ask for extra-credit work to raise his grade. In his career, he shone because of his diligence and the long hours he put in. He was skillful in court and often succeeded in suing for his clients' rights. But when he lost a case, he blamed himself. Surely there was a better argument he could have made. He would then review the transcripts of the court appearance, combing through them for any possible error he had made.

After a while the stress of his work started taking a toll. Kebede was exhausted physically from all the extra hours he put in, he felt burdened by the feelings of responsibility he assumed for his clients' well-being, and he was mentally drained by his constant self-criticism. He noticed he was caring a little less about his clients and started to feel disconnected from them. Eventually he began to dread going to the office.

HOW PERFECTIONISM CONTRIBUTES TO BURNOUT

Perfectionism is a personality trait defined by the tendency to strive for flawlessness, set unrealistically high standards for oneself, and become self-critical when these high standards aren't met. Research shows that if you're a perfectionist, you're vulnerable to burnout for several reasons. First, you're highly committed to whatever you put your mind to. Although being dedicated is admirable, perfectionists often overcommit. You may invest excessive time and effort into tasks and projects to get things right, often at the expense of your personal life. When perfectionists like Kebede take on more responsibility than is reasonable, they end up working crazy hours to meet those responsibilities. Essential acts of self-care such as eating well, exercising, sleeping, and spending time with friends can fall by the wayside. Eventually the body gives out in exhaustion and burnout sets in.

It's not just physical exhaustion that plagues perfectionists. When you have unrealistically high standards, the pressure to meet self-imposed demands mentally drains you too. Even very good isn't good enough; only perfection will do. It's already stressful to do a difficult job, but even more stressful if the expectation is that you must do that difficult job flawlessly. With no wiggle room, you'll inevitably see yourself as falling short. Perfectionism can lead to an obsessive focus on detail and the desire to control every aspect of one's work. But none of us can control all the factors that determine whether our work will be successful—outside forces and unexpected occurrences always play a role. This means that even when you do everything right, perfectionism leaves you unhappy and dissatisfied with your achievements.

And when you don't do everything exactly right—in other words, when you make errors or poor choices (gasp!)—the response can be downright cruel. You may call yourself names and say mean things that you would never say to someone you cared about. Harsh self-criticism activates the fight/flight/freeze response, which generates additional physiological and psychological stress (more on self-criticism in the next chapter). The self-critical tendencies of perfectionists also backfire. The assumption is that being cruel to yourself after making mistakes will be so painful that you'll never do it again. But all it really does is spark anxiety and create feelings of inadequacy, shame, and eventually depression. All these factors make it more, not less, likely that you will make mistakes in the future.

> **You may think beating yourself up will help you be perfect, but it will make it harder to get things right.**

Finally, perfectionists suffer from fear of failure. If you don't accept failure of any kind, the very thought of potentially failing can send shivers down your spine. This creates constant worry that never abates. Fear of failure can also lead to procrastination: you put off those tasks that you might fail at because they're risky. This increases stress as deadlines loom and reduces the amount of time available to do tasks well.

Perfectionism is a sinkhole that drains your mental, emotional, and physical resources and sucks you into the pit called burnout. The extra attention you pay, the extra work you do, can certainly contribute to your success. But the unrealistic expectations, the excessive taking of responsibility, overwork, self-criticism, fear of failure, anxiety, and stress you experience make things much harder than they need to be.

ARE YOU A PERFECTIONIST?

- ☐ Do you often have the feeling that you're not good enough?
- ☐ Do you try to do everything as well as possible?
- ☐ Do you feel like you're only as good as your last achievement?
- ☐ Do you adopt unrealistically high standards for yourself?
- ☐ Do you beat yourself up for making small mistakes?
- ☐ Do you keep working harder and harder, despite feeling more and more exhausted?
- ☐ Are you afraid of failure?

PERFECTIONISM AND SELF-WORTH

Research shows that perfectionists tend to have what is called *contingent self-esteem*, meaning our sense of self-worth depends on achievement in those areas of life that are important to our identity. If being a competitive runner is key to your identity and you have contingent self-esteem, you will feel on top of the world if you win that next race but like a total loser if you come in third. (You probably won't mind if you lose a karaoke contest if you don't identify as a good singer.) Whether you're an ER nurse, a schoolteacher, or a child at your ill parent's bedside, if you're a perfectionist, you will feel good about yourself when you meet your high standards and bad about yourself when you don't.

Perfectionism is a false friend. We think that trying so hard will help us, but when we set unrealistic standards for ourselves and then judge ourselves harshly for not meeting them, we just end up shooting ourselves in the foot. Perfectionism is also a fair-weather friend. It provides a sense of worthiness in the good times but deserts us when we need it most, when we fail or fall short. For instance, Kebede would beam with pride and confidence when he won a case for a client but hang his head in shame the next week if he lost a case. His self-esteem bounced up and down like a yo-yo on a trampoline. This instability in self-worth left him more vulnerable to stress, anxiety, feelings of inadequacy, and depression—all contributors to burnout.

Self-compassion, on the other hand, is a true and stable friend. With self-compassion our sense of self-worth isn't contingent on success or failure; it's rooted in being a flawed human being doing the best we can in the moment. Self-compassion provides a source of unconditional self-worth that is always available, regardless of circumstances.

> **Perfectionism is a false and fickle friend. Self-compassion is a true and constant friend.**

DOES SELF-COMPASSION LOWER YOUR STANDARDS?

Self-compassion helps us let go of the idea that we are in complete control of how things turn out. The truth is, life happens. To be human means making mistakes, getting it wrong, and missing the mark. But if self-compassion says you're "good enough," doesn't that mean you'll set the bar too low and stop aiming for greatness?

Interestingly, studies show that self-compassionate people still set high standards for themselves: if you care about yourself, you will want to reach your goals and realize your dreams. The big difference is how self-compassionate people relate to themselves when they fail to meet their high standards. They are kind and supportive rather than cold and cutting toward themselves. With a sense of worth and self-confidence intact, and the safety that comes from knowing it's okay to fail, they are more likely to pick themselves up and try again. This orientation toward growth and learning contributes to success.

We recently conducted a study of how self-compassion training impacted NCAA athletes. In the United States, college players have incredibly high standards for themselves. Good enough means being damn good. College scholarships and future professional careers depend on excellence, and slacking means being kicked off the team. We found that athletes who learned to be compassionate toward their mistakes in games or shortcomings in their training routines became less self-critical and experienced reductions in depression, anxiety, and stress. Most telling, they reported that their athletic performance improved and their coaches agreed with this assessment. Being kind to yourself doesn't mean letting your standards slip; it simply means you have more resources available to meet them.

GIVING YOURSELF COMPASSION FOR BEING A PERFECTIONIST

If you're a perfectionist, by now you might be interpreting your perfectionism as a sign of being imperfect. And since you're probably a burned-out perfectionist or you wouldn't be reading this book, you're probably also down on yourself for contributing to your exhausted state. First, it's important to be kind to yourself for striving so hard. You're trying desperately to do good work here. Also, no one consciously chooses to be a perfectionist. Perfectionism is typically a learned behavior stemming from pain in our childhood. People who grew up with parents or other adults who were highly critical or demanding learned that when their performance was perfect, they were safe. If we don't do anything wrong, we can't be criticized. This pattern typically starts with fear of criticism from parents, teachers, and others who have some authority over us and eventually becomes internalized.

This is certainly what happened with Kebede. He loved his father and greatly respected him, and his approval felt essential to Kebede's survival. It killed him to see that look of disappointment cloud his father's face when Kebede's grades weren't perfect. He assumed that his father would stop loving him if he didn't excel in all his classes. Even though that probably wasn't true, Kebede wasn't going to risk it. The pain of working long hours and studying till he dropped was not as bad as the pain of disappointing Dad. At some point Kebede came to rely on perfectionism to make his way in the world. And that was a very human thing to do.

We can be kind and understanding to ourselves for patterns of perfectionism, but at the same time, caring about ourselves means trying to do something different. Perfectionism isn't helping us, and it's contributing to our feelings of burnout. We can learn a different approach to our work that will be more effective and less exhausting: self-compassion.

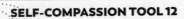

SELF-COMPASSION TOOL 12
Letting Go of the Need to Be Perfect

Even if we don't have the personality trait of perfectionism, we all want to get things right. Because we receive so many messages in our society that we need to achieve in the work realm to be worthy, it can be challenging to let go of the need to be perfect in those areas of life that are important to us. See if this writing exercise can help.

✦ Think about some aspect of your work life where perfectionism may be rearing its head. For instance, maybe you expect yourself to answer every email in a timely manner. Maybe you're a caregiver and you expect to fully meet the needs of the person you're caring for. Maybe you're an accountant who expects that you will never make a miscalculation in your balance sheets. Please focus on an area of your work that's important, but not crucial to the safety of yourself or others (for instance, a doctor who expects not to make a mistake while performing open-heart surgery). Focus on one way in which you're being perfectionistic.

✦ Imagine that you fail to meet your expectations or you make a mistake in this area of your work life. What are you afraid might happen to you?

✦ Notice whether you're focused on how your work performance will be affected (for example, it will slow you down) or on what it says about you (you'll be a laughingstock, embarrassed, a failure).

✦ What emotions come up for you when you imagine not meeting your expectations? Fear, anxiety, stress, shame, disappointment, sadness, frustration, anger?

✦ If it feels comfortable, take two or three deep breaths and put your hand on your heart or some other soothing place. Allow yourself to get in touch with any discomfort in your body.

✦ Now speak to yourself (out loud or silently) in warm, compassionate language about the desire to be perfect. You might imagine what you would say to a friend who was causing themselves unnecessary stress and tension due to perfectionism or what a good friend might say to you. Try something like: "It's okay to be imperfect and make mistakes." "You're only human." "Your worth doesn't depend on success." "I love you unconditionally."

✦ If feelings of fear and anxiety are especially strong, you can give assurances to yourself like "I'm here for you. I won't abandon you. Just do the best you can and take it step by step."

✦ Finally, try to let yourself be as you are, flawed and imperfect. Realize that you are not alone, that your imperfections are what make you a card-carrying member of the human race.

When Kebede did this exercise, he got very emotional. He focused on his unrealistic expectation that he could win all his court cases. The truth was that he won plenty, but when he didn't succeed it tore him up inside. When he thought about the impact of failing, he realized that his focus was primarily on what it said about him. He cared about his clients, of course, but what upset him the most was the look on their faces when he had to tell them he had lost their case. He felt ineffective and incompetent. Feelings of shame arose. He imagined the face of his dad as a newly arrived immigrant being deeply disappointed in him.

So Kebede gently placed his hands on his heart and held himself while feeling his discomfort. The warmth of his hands felt supportive. He allowed the pain in, and tears started forming in his eyes.

At first when he said "It's okay to be imperfect" and "Your worth doesn't depend on success," he didn't believe it. But then he imagined that one of his colleagues at the law firm came to him with similar feelings of shame over not winning a case. Without hesitation he would say "You can't control everything; you're only human. Losing comes with the territory. Don't be so hard on yourself." When he imagined that his colleague said these words back to him, he could receive the words more easily. He saw the truth of them.

Kebede started to practice being more compassionate to himself at work and setting more realistic expectations, and he noticed his stress started to diminish. He stopped working such crazy hours and spent more time on doing those things that replenished him. What filled his cup the most was knowing that his worth was unconditional. That he didn't have to earn it and that it was okay to be imperfect.

Self-compassion allows us to embrace our imperfections and realize that our flawed humanity is what connects us to others. What a relief. Although self-compassion won't magically make your burnout disappear, it can be a crucial pressure-release valve for the stress caused by perfectionism. Once you aren't so anxious and exhausted, and once you know that you'll catch yourself if you fall, it will become easier to recover from burnout.

Although perfectionists are especially self-critical, self-criticism is a feature of life for everyone, perfectionistic or not. There are powerful reasons why our inner critic speaks so loudly, which we examine in the next chapter.

WHY WE BEAT OURSELVES UP

Understanding the Inner Critic

Have you ever called yourself weak and worthless for not having an ounce of energy left to do your work? Or felt like you needed to mentally slap yourself to get going? Have you heard a stern voice that says you should be stronger, more resilient, hardworking, dedicated, or selfless? We often beat ourselves up for feeling beaten down. We think there must be something wrong with us for feeling so tired and depleted. But when we criticize ourselves for being burned out, we just end up feeling more wiped out and more burned out.

This self-critical voice probably isn't new. In fact, it likely played a role in your becoming burned out in the first place. As described in the last chapter, the qualities that make us vulnerable to burnout—including caring deeply about our work and valuing self-sacrifice—often lead us to set very high standards for ourselves. We use self-criticism as an engine of action, spurring us to try harder and do better, to keep going for as long as we can. Metaphorically we put our own head on the chopping block and relentlessly threaten ourselves with the worst fate—viewing ourselves as failures—so that we won't be complacent. By doing so, we drain even more of the resources we need to keep going.

Self-criticism causes the same physiological changes as any other chronic stressor. It elevates cortisol levels, leading to hypertension and even cardiovascular disease. It's also a major cause of depression, as the mind shuts down in response to chronic self-attack. Self-criticism deflates us as surely as a nail punctures a tire.

HOW SELF-CRITICAL ARE YOU?

❑ When something goes wrong, do you quickly point the finger of blame at yourself?

❑ Do you feel ashamed when you come up short on knowledge or skill?

❑ Do you scold yourself to try to improve your performance?

❑ Do you harshly judge yourself or your work?

❑ Do you negatively compare yourself to others?

❑ Do you call yourself demeaning names when you make a mistake?

Mei recently completed medical school at a prestigious university and is doing her residency at the university's clinic. She has just been appointed chief resident, and her parents couldn't be prouder. This appointment represents one of the final stepping stones in a journey that has demanded years of laser focus and grueling hours. It's a great honor to be chief resident, but now that Mei has added so much work on top of her own training—clinical scheduling, planning conferences, and helping other residents resolve grievances with the university faculty—the word *grueling* has taken on new meaning. The other residents at the clinic have no idea of the weight she's carrying. They see a stalwart advocate with a wicked sense of humor that can skewer "difficult" faculty members and attending physicians. They don't know that the person Mei skewers most is herself.

Mei often walks the halls with her head down, silently castigating herself for not being up to the task of her new role. She's been procrastinating on studying for her medical board certification exams, which are coming up in six months. She can't sleep at night, even as exhausted as she is, agonizing over how overwhelmed she feels. Her mind spins, worried that she doesn't have what it takes to be a successful doctor, that she might fail her whole family if she doesn't "step up." She wakes up with a racing heart, in terror that this will finally be the day she'll be exposed as an incompetent fraud. But instead of reconsidering her strategy of self-criticism, she doubles down on it.

WHY DO WE DO IT?

We all have a part of ourselves that we call "the inner critic." For some this critic is harsh and belittling, and for others it's more of a quiet feeling of shame or disappointment. Our inner tyrant may have emerged when we were young children or a bit later, but by adulthood most of us are very familiar with its disparaging voice. Self-criticism doesn't feel pleasant, so why would we volunteer to torment ourselves? Because at some level we think it's good for us. We think self-criticism helps motivate us to improve. In fact, research shows that the biggest block to self-compassion is the belief it will undermine our motivation.

Consciously or unconsciously, we believe we need a hard kick in the butt to reach our goals, whether it's getting through graduate school, impressing the boss, being more effective with clients, or getting Dad to his medical appointments on time. This belief isn't completely ill-founded: harsh criticism sometimes gets results. Maybe in the past you successfully berated yourself into pulling an all-nighter so you'd be prepared for that big meeting in the morning or shamed yourself out of bed to soothe a colicky infant for the fourth time in a single night. But self-criticism comes with a hefty price tag and has negative side effects.

Imagine using harsh criticism to motivate a child you're trying to teach to ride a bike. The child hops on and falls off, tries again, and falls down even harder. Now imagine that you make fun of the kid and call them a clumsy, incompetent loser. This approach might work. They'll get the message that you won't respect them until they get it right. Several scraped knees and bruised elbows later, the kid may figure it out. But have you made it easier for the child or harder? Feeling upset, ashamed, and stupid doesn't exactly put anyone in the right mental state to learn a new skill. And if the child doesn't figure out the bike on their own, they're likely to stop trying and give up altogether. Research shows that self-criticism has the same effect. It increases anxiety, undermines self-confidence, creates fear of failure, and makes it harder to learn from mistakes. It is also directly tied to shame, depression, and suicidal ideation—hardly the best get-up-and-go mind states.

A much more effective approach with the child would be to show them compassion and kindness when they fall off the bike. You could help them up and give them a hug, reassuring them that it's okay to fall—that's how we learn! Warmth, understanding, and useful tips on how to keep one's balance will increase the child's ability to master the skill. The same applies with self-compassionate motivation (see Chapter 18), so why don't we make the better choice?

A Ploy for Safety

The underlying intent of our inner critic is a good one: it's simply trying to keep us safe. When we see a problem in ourselves or our environment or feel threatened in any way, the fight/flight/freeze response is activated and turns inward. We castigate ourselves, hoping that we'll coerce ourselves into doing better so that we'll avoid failing and *be safe*. We flee into feelings of shame and isolation to avoid the judgment and criticism of others (beating them to the punch, so to speak) so that we'll *be safe*. We freeze and ruminate, hoping that maybe after rolling our problems around in our head for the sixty-seventh time we'll figure out a solution and *be safe*. We don't want to criticize ourselves for criticizing ourselves, because that mean voice in our heads is actually trying to protect us. It's just not very good at it.

One of the things self-criticism gives us is a sense of power and control. The inner critic stands tall, with complete certitude of being correct. It feels better to say we *should* have gotten it right—which presumes that we *could* have gotten it right if we had tried hard enough—than to acknowledge that sometimes, try as we might, we come up short. Although this sense of control is an illusion, it's easy to see why we cling to it in a bid for safety.

> **As painful as self-criticism feels, its intention is good: it's trying to keep us safe.**

Self-criticism may also have served us as children. For some people the inner critic represents the internalized critical or shaming messages of parents or other caregivers. Children's survival depends on trusting what the adults in their lives tell them. A kid can't say to a critical adult "You're wrong! I'm okay exactly as I am." Not only would it make the adult angry, but it would be frightening to think adults don't know what they're talking about. Children rely on adults for guidance and all the other necessities of life. Research suggests that children not only internalize the critical messages parents direct at them personally, they also internalize their parents' own self-critical messages. When kids hear their parents reproaching themselves for making mistakes, they learn that this is the "right" way to talk to themselves.

As we become adults ourselves, however, self-criticism is clearly no longer keeping us safe. It's making things worse by undermining our ability to give ourselves compassion and support, especially when faced with a challenge as daunting as recovering from burnout.

The Inner Critic Has a Role to Play

Once you recognize the harm that your inner critic is doing, it might be tempting to want to get rid of it. However, the inner critic is playing an important role: it perceives a danger and is trying to warn you about it. If you try to shut it down, it will just scream louder. There is a highly effective therapy model called *internal family systems* (IFS) that views the inner critic as a part of ourselves that is interacting with other parts of ourselves (just like different members of a family, but all operating in our own minds). We've found this model very useful in working effectively with the inner critic, and in fact it's useful for understanding how we relate to burnout in general.

The idea is that there are certain clusters of thoughts/emotions/behaviors inside us that we can call *parts*. These parts often form when we're young and relatively immature. We have hidden parts that carry the burden of scary and difficult emotions like shame, fear, hurt, and grief. We also have protector parts with the job of keeping us safe, largely by preventing ourselves from feeling these scary emotions. Protectors may be angry and defensive toward others, but they can also be inner critics that use judgment and disapproval to keep us in line or get us moving.

When a particular part is triggered by life circumstances, or perhaps a thought or feeling, our awareness often becomes completely overtaken by it. When your "incompetent" part is triggered, you get lost in feelings of shame and unworthiness. When your warrior part is triggered, you become consumed by anger and rigidly convinced that others are in the wrong. When your inner critic is triggered, you believe the only way to get things right is to be harsh and cruel to yourself.

LISTENING TO OUR COMPASSIONATE SELF

Albert Einstein, when discussing the implications of the atomic bomb, stressed that we can't solve a problem with the same mind that created it. We need to step out of our immature parts so that we aren't limited by their simplistic perspectives. Fortunately, we also have a part of us that is wise and mature that can come to our aid. You can think of this as your higher self, your spiritual self, your compassionate self, or if you're more scientifically oriented, your mammalian care-giving system.

When we take the perspective of our compassionate self as we relate to our other parts, we're able to disentangle from them. Instead of being lost in self-criticism, for instance, we can be curious about our inner critic in a kind and friendly way. Our inner critic then feels heard and doesn't have to shout so loudly to warn us of danger. This allows us to tune in to our compassionate self, who can see the larger picture of what's happening with more wisdom and complexity. And its methods are more effective in spurring growth and change than beating ourselves over the head.

When our compassionate self is kind and curious about our inner critic, our critical voice doesn't shout so loudly.

It's hard to feel inspired to do anything when we're burned out, but when our inner critic is in the driver's seat, it's even harder. The following exercise is based on IFS principles and is one that we use in the MSC program to help people understand their inner critic, find the voice of their inner compassionate self, and make change from a wiser and kinder perspective.

SELF-COMPASSION TOOL 13
Finding Your Compassionate Voice

This written exercise explores the voice of your inner critic. If you know your inner critic is the internalized voice of someone in your past who was abusive, or if intrusive memories come up during the exercise, please skip this practice. You can work through it later when you feel strong and ready, or perhaps with the help of a therapist.

✦ Think about a *behavior* you would like to change that's related to your feelings of burnout. Choose one that's causing problems for you but is mildly to moderately problematic, not extremely harmful (like abusing drugs). Maybe you're so exhausted you're having trouble getting out of bed in the morning and it's making you late to work. Or maybe you're so stressed you're snapping at your kids and it's starting to impact them. Please write down the burnout-related behavior you would like to change as well as the problems it's causing in your life.

Identifying the Inner Critic

✦ Write down how you typically react when you find yourself engaging in this behavior. How does your inner critic express itself? With unkind words? A particular harsh tone? With a sense of coldness or disappointment or perhaps a felt sense in the body?

Compassion for Feeling Criticized

✦ Take a moment to get in touch with the part of yourself that feels criticized. How does it feel to receive this message, and what is its impact on you?

✦ Try writing a few words of compassion for how hard it is to receive this harsh treatment—perhaps by validating your emotions: "I'm sorry you've experienced this. It's been so hard and painful for you."

Turning toward Your Inner Critic

✦ Now try to turn toward your inner critic with interest and curiosity. Reflect for a moment on *why* the criticism has gone on for so long. Is the inner critic trying to protect you in some way, to keep you safe from danger, or to help you—even if the result has been unproductive? If so, please write down what the inner critic may be trying to do for you.

✦ If you can't find any way that your inner critic is trying to help you, or you realize it's the internalized voice of someone abusive from your past, please skip the next step and continue to give yourself compassion for the pain of self-criticism.

✦ If you did identify a way your inner critic is trying to help you, however, see if you can acknowledge its efforts by writing down a few words of thanks. Let your inner critic know that even though it may not be serving you very well now, its intention was good and it was doing its best. You might also express some compassion for the difficult task and negative feelings experienced by the inner critic, perhaps for many years.

Finding Your Compassionate Self

✦ Now that the inner critic has been acknowledged, you're going to switch perspectives and make some space for the voice of your compassionate self.

✦ This part of yourself loves and accepts you unconditionally. However, your compassionate self also recognizes how the behavior you criticize yourself for is contributing to your burnout. It wants you to change—as the inner critic does—but for very different reasons.

✦ Please put your hands over your heart or another soothing place, feeling their warmth. Allow your compassionate self to emerge, perhaps as an image, a posture, or simply a loving feeling.

✦ Reflect again on the behavior you struggle with. Your compassionate self would like you to try to make a change—not because you're unacceptable as you are, but because it wants the best for you. It doesn't want you to suffer due to this behavior any longer.

✦ If you're having trouble getting in touch with your compassionate self, you can also bring to mind an image of a person who cares deeply about you (like a friend or grandparent) or an ideal image that represents compassion to you.

✦ Start to write a little letter to yourself in a compassionate voice, freely and spontaneously, addressing the behavior you would like to change. What words of wisdom, understanding, and encouragement spring from this deep desire for your well-being?

✦ If you're struggling to find words, it might be easier to consider what you would say to a dear friend who struggled with the same issue as you or what that friend would say to you.

✦ If you managed to write a few compassionate words to yourself, see if you can reread them and savor the feeling of those words flowing from your own hand. If you had difficulty finding compassionate words, that's okay too. It takes some time. The important thing is that we set our intention to try to be kinder to ourselves, and eventually new habits will form.

This exercise had a big impact on Mei. She had chosen procrastination on her board exams as her problematic behavior. It was easy to identify how her inner critic showed up for this one. "You're so stupid. Why did you accept the position of chief resident when you can't study and fulfill your duties at the same time? You've got a big head, and you're also lazy. You'll never pass your exams, especially at this rate." Recognizing that her inner critic was trying to protect her from failure was a game changer. Mei had thought of her inner critic as a cruel despot that was cold and mean, and she often criticized herself for being so self-critical. But when she asked herself if the inner critic was trying to keep her safe, the answer was clear: of course it was. It was trying to drive her forward, to prevent complacency and keep her humble.

Mei also saw that she had internalized these messages from her parents when growing up, who often criticized themselves in order to work harder. When Mei thanked her inner critic for its efforts to help, she felt her inner critic relax inside.

What really impressed Mei, however, was what her compassionate self said once her inner critic felt validated. This caring voice wouldn't let her slide on study time, because that wouldn't be kind. Instead, it gave her wise advice about how to manage her time better to reach her goals: saying no to residents' requests for help that weren't directly related to her job as chief resident; being encouraging toward herself when reviewing her day so she slept better and got some early-morning study time. Feeling supported in this way helped her feel more confident that she was up to the task.

When we get burned out, we're often extremely hard on ourselves. But we can treat our tendency toward self-criticism—this inborn safety behavior—with compassion. It's often a young, innocent part of ourselves that only knows how to bully to prevent harm. While people may worry that self-compassion will undermine their drive, love and kindness are a more effective engine of growth and change than fear.

Our compassionate self isn't interested only in change on the inside; it's also interested in change on the outside. Many of the factors leading to burnout stem from the external circumstances of our lives: broken systems, unfair working conditions, or people crossing boundaries. The next chapter dives into how taking action with fierce self-compassion can help us address some of the situational factors causing burnout.

14

DOING SOMETHING ABOUT IT

Fierce Self-Compassion in Action

Self-compassion can be a lifesaver when we're burned out. When we accept ourselves and validate our feelings of exhaustion and hopelessness, healing can begin. But acceptance alone can't reverse burnout. When we tell ourselves that "it's only natural to feel this way," we often find ourselves completing the sentence with "because my job sucks!" We can't just soothe ourselves and expect our job to become less sucky.

Burnout is not only about our internal emotional experience. It also springs from the demands placed on us by our employers or the environments in which we work. Unreasonable demands may be made on our time. Resources are often stretched, companies understaffed, and in far too many cases the almighty dollar takes precedence over workers' health and welfare. People can become exhausted by circumstances of greed or incompetence or unfairness even more than they are by self-criticism and perfectionism.

For instance, Annabelle isn't given the respect she deserves. She started as a bookkeeper at her accounting firm ten years ago but took evening courses at an online school so she could pass the CPA exam and is now officially an accountant. But the other accountants at her firm still treat Annabelle as an assistant rather than a colleague, routinely asking her to make coffee or photocopies. Her boss also gives her lots of grunt work, assigning her low-level projects that don't require creative problem solving. Since Annabelle was promoted, she's been expected to work longer hours, but the pay raise she received isn't commensurate with her new title. The situation has left her feeling disgruntled and burned out.

Annabelle is generally a kind person—to herself as well as others. She doesn't cut herself down or shame herself. Her biggest challenge is that she's afraid to speak to her colleagues about their insensitive requests or ask her boss for more pay, better working hours, or a more varied caseload. Annabelle tends to just dismiss it. "It's no big deal," she tells herself. "It will probably get better over time." Meanwhile deep down she's simmering with resentment, which is adding to her exhaustion.

Annabelle was raised in a traditional household where women who spoke up or who were too assertive were dismissed as ill-tempered shrews. She was taught that a woman is valued for being sweet and cheerful. Annabelle internalized the belief that she should never raise her voice or (God forbid) get angry. She was supposed to smooth things over, not make waves. This narrow view of acceptable feminine behavior cut Annabelle off from her inner strength and power.

As Annabelle would eventually come to learn, compassion isn't just about acceptance; it's also about taking action to fight for what's right. Fierce self-compassion helps us address the situational causes of burnout by spurring us to speak up, say no, draw boundaries, end injustice, or make changes. To alleviate suffering, we must focus on improving the circumstances of our lives and fix what's broken on the outside as well as inside.

FINDING OUR INNER MAMA BEAR

Fierce self-compassion feels quite different than tender self-compassion, which has a soft and nurturing quality. Metaphorically speaking, tender self-compassion is like a loving parent caring for a crying child. Warm acceptance allows us to calm down and helps us feel loved and worthy. In contrast, fierce self-compassion has a powerful and energetic quality, more like a Mama Bear who ferociously protects her cubs from harm, travels miles to find food for them, and eventually boots them out of the den when they're ready to fend for themselves. Fierce self-compassion spurs us to action so that we protect, provide for, and motivate ourselves. We don't have to be a parent or identify as female to find our inner Mama Bear. It's a universal energy that's ready to fight for us, meet our needs, and get us moving whenever we need it.

Fierce self-compassion is about taking action to protect ourselves, provide for our needs, and motivate change.

A nurse who took our eight-week Fierce Self-Compassion course at the Center for Mindful Self-Compassion told us how the course had strengthened her backbone. One day, in a packed and chaotic emergency room, she bravely stood up for herself. As patients waited for hours with little information on when they'd be seen, a man pointed to her sitting at her desk beyond the waiting room and loudly accused her of "hiding behind that window" and not caring about them. She calmly entered the waiting room with her back tall and replied with dignity, "I'm not hiding, I'm doing my work. Yes, this is a problem. I apologize. The system is broken and we're understaffed. I understand your frustration. I'm frustrated too. Please, call the hospital administration, your local politicians, anyone you can think of, and tell them about this. The system is broken. We're doing the best we can."

Clearly this nurse felt as depleted and helpless as anyone. But she was not only able to keep working, she was also able to speak out about the real problems at her hospital. Who knows if anyone in that waiting room really heard her or ever made a call, but she felt better just for expressing herself and taking a small step toward change.

Might you do the same? You may be too burned out to attempt big changes to the structural causes of burnout. But can you think of one small, doable step that might help?

- ☐ Could you propose more realistic deadlines to your supervisor?
- ☐ Suggest rotating fifteen-minute breaks among staff?
- ☐ Try reducing your work hours by ten percent?
- ☐ Speak up about feeling that you're being treated unfairly?
- ☐ Perhaps write a letter to a local politician?
- ☐ Maybe ask a neighbor to come sit with an elderly parent for an hour in the evening?
- ☐ Could you (fill in the blank with your own creative ideas)?

FIERCE AND TENDER SELF-COMPASSION: A FORMIDABLE DUO

We need both fierce and tender self-compassion to counteract burnout. It's like yin and yang—an imbalance between these two energies isn't healthy. If we're too accepting of our feelings of exhaustion without fierce action to address their external causes, broken systems will never change. But if we're too fierce without tenderness toward ourselves and our emotions, we'll just stress and exhaust ourselves further.

To find balance, we need to honor and invite both energies to arise, merging and integrating within us. We can ask simple questions like "Where in my life do I need to find more courage to speak up, say no, take action?" and "Where in my life do I need to be more accepting of myself or others as human beings doing the best we can in the moment?" If you start a petition against unfair policies at work, for instance, can you hold your pain with warmth while remembering that those creating the policies are human beings also worthy of consideration?

Combining and balancing the energies of fierce and tender self-compassion creates a type of caring force that can make real change in the world. As Martin Luther King Jr. wrote, "Power without love is reckless and abusive, and love without power is sentimental and anemic. Power at its best is love implementing the demands of justice, and justice at its best is power correcting everything that stands against love."

ANGER AS AN ENERGIZING ALLY

Sometimes anger gets a bad rap, especially in the mindfulness and compassion world. But anger has a role to play in fierce self-compassion. It's a natural emotion that evolved for a purpose: to alert us to threats so we can protect ourselves or those we care about. Anger energizes us and provides a sense of empowerment. It overrides our fear response and boosts our courage. It also serves an important expressive function by clearly pointing out—to both ourselves and others—that something is wrong. Although venting and ruminating on anger is problematic, it can be cathartic in some circumstances, like swearing after stubbing a toe (and research shows doing so reduces perceived pain!).

Getting angry at the causes of burnout—inadequate pay, rude remarks, impossible deadlines, a cold and impersonal system (the list goes on)—may be useful when the anger is constructive and harnessed for good. Being pissed off about an unfair work situation, for instance, may motivate you to speak up or make a change. As long as you don't attack people personally and aren't insulting or demeaning, your anger serves an important purpose: it clearly communicates

> ### Constructive versus Destructive Anger
>
> **Anger can be constructive or destructive, depending on whether it prevents or causes harm.**
>
> ✦ Constructive anger is a benevolent energy that focuses on protection; destructive anger is a hostile energy that seeks to retaliate and destroy.
>
> ✦ Constructive anger focuses on behaviors or situations; destructive anger is personal and dehumanizes others.
>
> ✦ Constructive anger is clear and sensitive to consequences; destructive anger is reactive and does not consider impacts on others.
>
> ✦ Constructive anger comes from love and the desire for well-being; destructive anger comes from fear and ego protection.

that you mean business. It can also give you the energy boost you need when you're so burned out that it feels impossible to get off the couch.

FIERCE SELF-COMPASSION IN ACTION

If we look at the three components of self-compassion in their fierce protective form, they are expressed as *brave, empowered clarity.*

Kindness inspires us to be brave and courageous so that we can take risks and act to improve our situation. It requires gumption and determination—like when we go on strike or ask for a raise. It may feel safer to stay at a toxic job or to ignore that cutting comment by a colleague or to surrender to an inefficient system that requires unnecessary work, but inaction is a form of self-harm. Kindness compels us to do whatever we can to help ourselves. This may take the form of drawing boundaries (more on this in Chapter 15), having difficult conversations, making a formal complaint to someone who has the authority to alter standard procedures, get help from others, or even change our job if possible.

Common humanity in its fierce form strengthens and empowers us. The feeling of connection reminds us that we aren't alone in the experience of burnout. We relate to those in situations similar to ours—parents of children with special needs, ER nurses, veterinarians, caregivers for elderly parents, firefighters, and others—and remember that many of our fellows are also burned out. Standing up for ourselves means standing up for them too. There is strength in numbers. When we forget this and feel isolated, we feel helpless. But when we bond with others, either in reality or simply mentally, we claim the human right to be well and whole and feel more inspired to act.

Finally, mindfulness allows us to see our problems clearly. We don't turn away from the truth if we've been treated unfairly or if things aren't working. Sometimes it's easier to downplay the gravity of our situation so that we don't have to expend energy to do something about it. This can be the case especially when we're exhausted and burned out. But if we don't acknowledge there's a problem, how are we ever going to fix it? Even if we can't do much to change our situation, it's important to be honest with ourselves and see clearly when harm is being done. At least this way we don't buy into the excuses.

> **Fierce self-compassion allows us to see our problems clearly, feel empowered by our sense of connection to others, and find the courage to act.**

For some people, especially those socialized as women, fierce self-compassion can feel uncomfortable and alien. But even if your inner Mama Bear is sleeping, it's still a part of your nature. With practice, you can wake from hibernation and claim your right to fair treatment. We've developed a version of the self-compassion break (introduced in Chapter 6) that's designed to evoke brave, empowered clarity when we need to take action to fight the causes of burnout. Why not give it a try?

SELF-COMPASSION TOOL 14
Protective Self-Compassion Break

Here is a practice that can help you develop your fierce self-compassion muscles, especially when you need to speak up or protect yourself in some way. You can use it at work or at home, and it takes only a few minutes. If you encounter a situation where you know that you need to stand up for yourself or take action against injustice, doing this practice can help strengthen your energy and resolve.

✦ Think of a situation in your life that is calling for the fierce energy of protection. Maybe a client is disrespectful of your time, or you are being treated unfairly by upper management, or your siblings are expecting you to provide all the care for your elderly parents, or something is happening at your workplace that is unjust or broken. Please choose a situation where you feel mild to moderately angry or threatened but not overwhelmed.

✦ Call up the situation in your mind's eye. What's happening? What's going on? Allow yourself to feel whatever emotions are arising. Fear, contempt, frustration?

✦ Make contact with the discomfort as a physical sensation and feel your body.

✦ Now try to adopt the attitude of Mama Bear. Sit tall, with your back straight, and roll your shoulders back.

✦ The first phrase evokes mindfulness—we see things clearly as they are. Try saying to yourself, slowly and with conviction: "My eyes are open." Other options are "I see the truth of what's happening" or "I will try to see this situation as clearly as possible."

✦ The second phrase focuses on common humanity. You remember your connection to something larger than yourself, allowing this recognition to empower you. Try saying, "I do not stand alone, I stand with others." Other options include "All human beings deserve just treatment" and "Me too."

✦ Now put a fist over your heart, as a gesture of fortitude and determination.

✦ The third phrase expresses self-kindness in the form of courage. Try saying with conviction: "I will be brave and strong." Another option might be "I will find my voice" or simply "No!"

✦ Imagine that someone you really cared about was being mistreated in a similar way. What would you say to this person to help them be strong, to speak up, to have fortitude? Now, can you offer the same message to yourself?

✦ Finally, put your other hand over your fist and hold it tenderly. The invitation is to combine the fierce energy of brave, empowered clarity with the tender energy of loving, connected presence. Give yourself full permission to feel the force of your power, your resolve, your truth, but to also be in touch with your natural caring.

✦ Aim your fierce compassion at the situations or behaviors causing harm, not at the person or people causing harm. They are human and you are human. Can you commit to taking action while still keeping the thread of love alive?

✦ See if you can allow both energies to flow.

When Annabelle first learned the protective self-compassion break, she felt uncomfortable. It seemed so unladylike. But her prediction that things at work would "probably get better over time" was proving inaccurate, and she realized if she never spoke up at the office, things would never change. She would never be respected by her colleagues or get the pay or interesting assignments she deserved. So every night she practiced.

Annabelle engaged mindfulness to see clearly how wrong it was for her colleagues to keep asking her to make copies and coffee. They should respect those long hours she spent to become a certified accountant! And it wasn't okay that she was underpaid and got all the grunt work! She stared this reality straight in the face.

Bringing in consideration of common humanity reminded Annabelle that many people were treated unfairly. This didn't diminish the importance of her situation, but it certainly helped her feel less alone. All over the world, people were up against it. She thought of all the "-isms"—racism, sexism, ageism, heterosexism, ableism, and so on. Speaking up for herself wasn't selfish; it was advancing the cause of justice. Remembering this made her feel more powerful.

Then Annabelle sat up straight and put her fist on her heart, embodying her inner Mama Bear. She dropped deep into her heart, and out of the depths of her being came a loud "NO! NO MORE!" She found her backbone. She found her anger—anger that had been suppressed throughout her life. She wouldn't stand for it any longer. She decided to talk to her boss and her work colleagues. This anger was something new for her, however, and it felt dangerous.

It really helped when she brought in some tenderness to balance the fierceness. No, she wasn't being treated fairly. Things had to change. But her boss and colleagues weren't bad people. They were also stressed and doing the best they could and probably didn't even think about how their behavior was impacting her. She could be strong and firm without being cold or mean. When she was able to feel tenderness and fierceness at the same time, Annabelle felt more authentic and complete.

After practicing every night for a week, Annabelle found the courage to make an appointment with her boss. She initiated a scary but ultimately rewarding conversation, pointing out how she was being treated differently from her colleagues. To her great surprise, her boss agreed with her and said she would try to rectify things. Wow. Even more gratifying, the next time her colleagues asked her to make coffee she said no. She told them that she was no longer the office assistant and didn't want to be treated as one. Her coworkers were caught off guard for sure, but they knew they were out of line. Two of them actually apologized. Annabelle grew to love this fierce Mama Bear side of herself, and she continued to give herself the respect she deserved.

What Annabelle did, especially with her colleagues, was draw a boundary. Drawing boundaries is essential to self-compassion but can be tricky and difficult to do. For this reason, in the next chapter we talk about how self-compassion can help us overcome some of the barriers that stand in the way of drawing effective boundaries.

15

DRAWING A LINE IN THE SAND

Learning How to Say No

How many times have you encountered the word *boundaries* lately? It's stamped all over workplace ethical codes and makes regular appearances in advice columns about how to succeed on the job and in personal relationships. And now that you're burned out, you might hear it in your head: "If only I had drawn firmer boundaries . . . "

A key aspect of dealing with burnout is knowing how to draw boundaries—when to decline requests for your time and energy or carve out space to meet your own needs. Boundaries also involve letting people know when their behavior is intrusive or unwanted. Drawing a line in the sand is complicated for everyone. In childhood, those who are agreeable and accommodating are given approval by parents and teachers, and this continues in adulthood with bosses, colleagues, and partners. It can be hard to disentangle one's sense of self-worth from being helpful or, in other words, compliant.

In fact, anyone trained to attend to the needs of others in their work, regardless of how they were socialized, can find drawing boundaries uncomfortable and stressful. When saying no sets off rumblings of uncertainty and fear, that sand (that you haven't drawn the line in) may turn to quicksand. When we don't draw boundaries, we give our time and energy away. When we don't say anything about someone's inappropriate behavior, we feel violated. This can turn into an exhausting downward spiral as the lack of boundaries makes us even more stressed.

Luis finds it difficult to draw boundaries. He's been working as a sales associate at a high-end men's clothing store for the last two years, and it's wearing him out. Luis is a young man with impeccable manners and a warm smile that makes everyone feel relaxed and welcome as soon as they walk in the door, from the nervous soon-to-be groom seeking a wedding suit to the demanding corporate boss wanting to impress at the upcoming summit. He deftly steers customers away from the unflattering or the wrong-for-the-occasion. He's deferential but never obsequious. He sells a whole lot of clothes, and his store manager loves him.

His colleagues also love him because he's so accommodating. He rarely says no to their requests, no matter how unreasonable: "Oh, Luis, do you mind clearing out the fitting rooms and putting everything back on the racks? I really need to get home." Or "Hey, buddy, you don't mind finishing out my shift, do you? I have a date tonight, and I can't be late. In fact, maybe you could give me some advice about what I should wear." Luis obliges with a tip of his head. He likes the fact that he's recognized as friendly and helpful. It feels good that everyone at the store appreciates and depends on him, including the manager and the customers. But these rewards come at a cost.

One day the dressing rooms were a complete disaster. It was high school prom, and a bunch of seniors swarmed through the store like a hurricane. He was supposed to close the store with another sales associate, but she said she wanted to leave early to go to a party. "You're cool, aren't you?" "Sure," Luis said with a fake smile. He wanted to be cool. As he was picking up the rumpled shirts and pants and jackets from the dressing room floor and putting them on hangers and organizing them on the racks by size, his stomach started churning. He collapsed in a chair and wanted to cry. He felt overwhelmed and exhausted by doing everyone else's job for them.

WHY WE HAVE TROUBLE SAYING NO

People who can't draw boundaries are ripe candidates for burnout. Why is it so hard to say no? Identifying the reasons for your discomfort can help you understand your patterns so that hopefully you can change them. Reluctance to say no may come from societal norms, the reactions of others, or our image of ourselves—sometimes a combination of all three.

'Tis Better to Give than Receive

Those in the helping and service professions (including personal caregivers) are highly susceptible to burnout, in part because self-sacrifice is written into the job description. These fields draw personalities that are naturally giving and generous, who reflexively say yes when asked to help. Another fundraiser? Sure, I can organize it (even though I work a fifty-hour week and have three young kids). Yes, I'll take on that extra shift (even though I'm exhausted and desperately need to sleep). It would be selfish to refuse, wouldn't it? And being selfish is the worst thing you can be if you identify as a caring and giving person.

The view of self-sacrifice as a noble virtue is culturally entrenched and typically unquestioned. It's worth looking at this notion more closely, however. The burden of self-sacrifice is not shared equally. Those on the bottom forgo their needs more often than those at the top. In fact, asymmetrical giving defines unequal power relationships. Those at the top portray self-sacrifice as noble to make this bitter truth more palatable and to manipulate the disenfranchised to willingly say yes when they have every right to say no.

People without power are led to believe it's noble to sacrifice themselves.

When we care about ourselves, we don't let ourselves be manipulated if we can help it. Fierce self-compassion spurs us to draw boundaries and say no because our needs count too. Research shows that self-compassionate people are less likely to subordinate their own needs to those of others. They don't prioritize their own needs either—they try to find compromise solutions that take everyone's needs into account. As Prentis Hemphill, CEO of the Embodiment Institute, has wisely said, "Boundaries are the distance at which I can love you and me simultaneously." This adage applies to work relationships as well as personal ones, although at work you might substitute the word *respect* for *love*.

Of course, there are situations in which self-sacrifice is appropriate: caring for children with chronic illnesses or other special needs, rushing to rescue someone trapped by a fire, staying up all night to get a foundation grant written by the morning deadline, or working two jobs to provide for one's family. What's not appropriate is the message that our worth is derived only from our usefulness to others. Saying yes as an authentic choice energizes us. Saying yes because we think we're *supposed* to say yes to be a good person drains us.

Fearing Others' Reactions

Even if we don't identify with self-sacrifice as a virtue, most of us are invested in what others think of us. Have you ever said yes to a request even though you really wanted to say no, so you would seem "nice"? Or kept quiet when someone acted inappropriately because you didn't want to be "rude"? This was certainly what drove Luis to cover for his work associates and agree to their unreasonable requests. He was so afraid of being disliked that he let others walk all over him.

The fear that people won't like us if we say no is not completely ill founded. Others *do* like us more when we do what they want us to do. But if we never risk displeasing them by saying no to requests for our time and energy, and we become drained and exhausted as a result, is it worth it? Others *do* like us more when we chuckle at their offensive jokes rather than calling them out. But if we don't speak up, our silence may be interpreted as validation and tacitly encourage bad behavior in the future. Again, is it worth it? Maybe it's better if others like us a little less and we like ourselves a little more. Instead of worrying about others' perception of us, maybe we should worry about whether we're healthy and fulfilled. If we're liked but stressed to the point where we can't get out of bed, we aren't helping anyone, least of all ourselves.

When we are self-compassionate, we aren't totally dependent on others' positive opinions. Our self-worth isn't contingent on social approval. This allows us to choose integrity over pleasing others. Fierce self-compassion gives us the strength and determination to say no when we need to and draw clear lines between behavior that we agree to and behavior that's unwanted. Tender self-compassion provides support and comfort if there are negative consequences for doing so. Self-compassion is the force that propels us to stay true to ourselves.

> **Self-compassion allows us to choose integrity over pleasing others.**

This is a nuanced issue, of course. Displeasing your friend who asks you to babysit is different from displeasing your boss who asks you to work late. As we mentioned, the ability to draw boundaries is intertwined with power dynamics. In the real world, none of us will be able to speak up or set the exact boundaries we want in every situation. You probably don't want to refuse a request to work weekends during a crunch time if you might be fired. Maybe the board meeting you're taking minutes for isn't the right place to call out the CEO's offensive comment. You may decide that even though you're sick of doing more than your share of household chores, it's not worth getting into yet another argument with your partner. *Only you can decide*. People living in poverty, the undereducated, and oppressed minority groups may not have the luxury of drawing boundaries if they are fighting for their very survival. These are real factors that need to be considered, and the last thing we want to do is beat ourselves up for not drawing adequate boundaries.

If we choose not to draw a boundary because the consequences would be too great, it's important that we know what we're doing and why. We need to be clear in our minds and hearts that we are valuable and worthy of getting our needs met and that we have the right to draw boundaries, even if we decide it's wisest not to do so right now. Unfortunately, all too often we fall into the trap of believing that we're less important than other people, that our needs and desires don't merit attention. Who am I to take time for myself, to rest, to play, to speak up, to express my opinion? When we buy into the idea sold to us by those with power and privilege, we dehumanize ourselves.

The truth is that every human being has the right to get their basic needs for protection and health and happiness met. With self-compassion we know what we deserve; we know our own value. So even if we choose not to draw a boundary in a particular instance, we retain the right to assert ourselves going forward when possible. Self-compassion requires wisdom when choosing how, when, where, and whether to draw boundaries so that our choice causes the least amount of suffering possible. It helps us determine whether drawing a boundary feels right or wrong, safe or unsafe, helpful or harmful.

DRAWING BOUNDARIES WITH CARING FORCE

The gentle, nurturing quality of tender self-compassion paves the way for us to be brave, take fierce action, and draw clear boundaries. It's important that these two faces of self-compassion be balanced and integrated. As with anger, if we say no in a way that's rude or insulting or demeans others, we're working against compassion. We need a strong back and a soft front (introduced in Chapter 10) so we can express ourselves firmly yet kindly. We want to maintain friendly relationships and respect others without sacrificing our needs or our truth. With practice, we can learn to be tactful, to say no while still respecting others' humanity along with our own. Only you can find the right language to demonstrate care for others as well as yourself, but self-compassionately asserting your boundaries might sound something like this:

- "I know this may disappoint you, but that's just not going to work for me right now."
- "I appreciate your asking me. I can't do it, but here are other options."
- "I would like to help, but I need to take care of myself by saying no."
- "You probably didn't mean to be offensive, but when you interrupted me, I felt like you weren't interested in what I had to say."
- "Each of us has a right to express our opinions, but I'd prefer it if we didn't discuss politics right now."

When we clearly and unequivocally speak up or say no (not hedging with responses like "Umm uhh, well . . . "), we can take a stand in a way that allows our voice to be heard. Drawing boundaries is an act of self-care. It models and reinforces the message that we're all ultimately responsible for our own well-being and that self-kindness means sometimes saying no. It also gives other people permission to do the same.

There are bookshelves full of advice on how to communicate boundaries effectively (the model of nonviolent communication developed by Marshall Rosenberg is particularly helpful). Our goal in this chapter is not so much to teach you *how* to draw boundaries, but rather to explore how self-compassion can help you let go of some of the barriers to this fierce action.

The following tool will help you explore your discomfort with drawing boundaries. You won't be focusing on drawing a boundary in your current life circumstances, given how complicated drawing boundaries is and how many variables there are to consider. Instead, you'll be asked to think of a past experience with drawing boundaries and consider how self-compassion may help you let go of limiting attitudes.

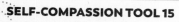

SELF-COMPASSION TOOL 15
Getting Comfortable with Boundaries

This is a writing exercise, so please take out a pen and paper or something else to write with.

✦ Think of a situation where you did *not* draw a boundary but wish you had. If you can, try to focus on a situation where the lack of a boundary contributed to your feelings of burnout. This could be something like agreeing to a coworker's request to take on work for them when your plate was already full; not saying anything when someone made rude remarks that stressed and upset you; or doing housework after a hard day's work even though your teenage child was supposed to do it. Please don't choose a traumatic situation, like someone being abusive, as feelings of overwhelm may make it harder for you to do the practice.

✦ Now ask yourself, "What prevented me from drawing the boundary I wanted to draw?"

- Were you worried about the consequences if you drew a boundary? If so, what did you think might happen?

- Did thoughts arise that stood in your way, such as "It wouldn't be nice to say no" or "I'd be excluded from the group" or "It would be selfish if I didn't help"?

- Did certain emotions stop you from drawing the boundary, such as fear, guilt, confusion, self-doubt?

✦ Try to give yourself some tender self-compassion for having done the best you could at the time and for whatever stood in the way of your drawing this boundary. Write a few words that validate and express understanding for what happened. What would you say to a good friend who was in a similar situation?

✦ Now see if you can call up some fierce protective energy. Sit up straight, roll your shoulders back, and imagine that fierce energy is flowing up and down your spine. Remind yourself that your needs are important too. You have the right to say no! It's okay to stand up for yourself! You don't have to always do what others want; you can also assert your own desires. Write some words of affirmation concerning your right to assert yourself.

✦ You might also consider these questions: Is it the end of the world if people don't like your decisions, if you're true to yourself? Does your self-worth depend on what other people think of you? Write whatever insights arise.

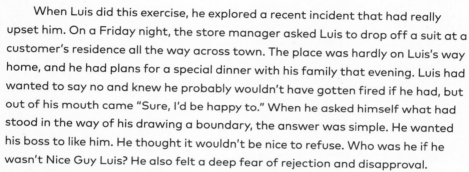

✦ Now imagine, if you could have done it differently, how you might have drawn that boundary. Could you imagine doing so in a way that was firm, wise, clear, and kind—that respected everyone's needs, including your own? Take a few moments to consider what you ideally might have done or said.

✦ Finally, how does it feel when you imagine having drawn this boundary? In particular, do you notice any difference in your feelings of burnout?

When Luis did this exercise, he explored a recent incident that had really upset him. On a Friday night, the store manager asked Luis to drop off a suit at a customer's residence all the way across town. The place was hardly on Luis's way home, and he had plans for a special dinner with his family that evening. Luis had wanted to say no and knew he probably wouldn't have gotten fired if he had, but out of his mouth came "Sure, I'd be happy to." When he asked himself what had stood in the way of his drawing a boundary, the answer was simple. He wanted his boss to like him. He thought it wouldn't be nice to refuse. Who was he if he wasn't Nice Guy Luis? He also felt a deep fear of rejection and disapproval.

At first Luis was ashamed for being such a coward. But then he gently put his hand on his heart and said, "I understand why it was so hard for you. You just want to be loved. Everyone wants to be loved and accepted. There's no shame in that." He immediately relaxed. It also felt good when he sat up straight and called in some fierce self-compassion. Luis said out loud, "I won't allow people to take advantage of my niceness anymore! I don't have to help everyone who asks. I'm a good and kind person. If other people don't like me as I am, that's their problem!"

Luis considered what he would have done differently if he could have. Or what he might do the next time a situation like this arose (which would probably be soon). Although it might have felt satisfying to say "Go f—— yourself," he knew that wasn't fair. His manager and colleagues were just trying to get their jobs done. Instead, maybe something straightforward like "I'd like to help, but I have a prior commitment—sorry about that" would have been enough. It was something Luis was going to have to experiment with. But when he imagined drawing a boundary, he was surprised at how much more energized and empowered he felt. His job was still tiring and demanding, but he suspected his feelings of burnout wouldn't be as strong once he stopped being a doormat and started being a door that he could choose to open and close according to his own will.

Self-compassion can help you value your authentic self so that you feel more comfortable speaking up and drawing boundaries. Especially when our work is difficult and draining, we need to guard our time and energy zealously, and this often means saying no. Another way that fierce self-compassion can help counter burnout is by enabling us to say yes—to ourselves. Asking ourselves what we need and taking action to fulfill our needs is a key aspect of self-care. In the next chapter, we examine how self-compassion can help us meet our own needs, starting with the fundamental ones essential to healing from burnout.

16

PROVIDING FOR OURSELVES

What Do I Need?

After you've created necessary boundaries—a fence around your garden—you'll have more emotional space to look around, see what might nourish you, and then decide what to plant. As adults, we must provide for ourselves because other people will never know precisely *what* we need, *when* we need it, and *how* to give it to us. Providing for ourselves isn't selfish; it's essential.

The first step toward providing for yourself is to determine what you need to be well. If you're feeling burned out and make that inquiry right now, does your answer resemble any of the following?

- "I need to stay at my computer until I get this report done!"
- "I need to make sure my daughter is comfortable before I can go to bed."
- "I need to find housing for these folks before I leave work, or they'll be on the street tonight!"

These answers are praiseworthy, but they don't reflect your needs. To begin with, there's a distinct lack of *you* in all of them. They all focus on *others'* needs—your boss's need for your report, your daughter's need for care, or your unhoused clients' need for a safe place to sleep. When the question about what we need defaults to what *others* need from us, we're on a path to burnout.

When we're *not* struggling, it can be uplifting to focus on the needs of others. Contributing to the lives of others can exponentially expand our joy. The

Dalai Lama describes compassion as "wise selfishness." Everyone benefits from kindness and generosity when it's freely given. But we must include ourselves in the circle of generosity and figure out how to care for others without abandoning ourselves in the process.

Winona, forty-three, is a single mother living in Albuquerque with her teenage daughter, Tallulah, who has Down syndrome. She knows what it's like to prioritize someone else's needs over her own and pay the price for it. Early on, Winona decided to give her daughter every opportunity to grow and thrive. She gave up her full-time job as a social worker and took part-time office work when Tallulah was young so she could care for her. It took every bit of Winona's free time, to say nothing of her modest savings. Whatever Tallulah wanted, Winona provided. For instance, Tallulah had a fascination for fancy hair clips—the more sparkly the better. Winona would spend hours tracking down pretty hair clips online and ordering them for Tallulah, even though they were sometimes expensive. She loved to see Tallulah's face light up with joy when a new clip arrived in the mail. Money was tight, however, and Winona was constantly stressed about paying her rent and utility bills.

Winona's doctor told her if she didn't watch her blood pressure, she was a prime candidate for heart disease despite her relatively young age. But in Winona's mind, being under pressure was a way of life. If she didn't feel exhausted at the end of the day, she felt she hadn't done enough for her daughter. Although Winona's generous heart was more than willing to keep pumping out the love, her anatomical heart was starting to give out.

Winona's friends noticed that she was running out of juice, but she dismissed their suggestions that she enroll Tallulah in a respite center run by a local charity for a week and take some time off. Tallulah wouldn't like that, she thought. She was the last person in the world to ask herself, "What do *I* need?"

THE QUINTESSENTIAL SELF-COMPASSION QUESTION

Compassion reflects the desire to alleviate suffering. Therefore, the quintessential *self*-compassion question is "What do I need?"

You don't have to ask "What do I need?" using those exact words, but you do require the curiosity and inclination of heart to discover what's ailing you and to consider what would help. When you're burned out, it's sometimes hard to know what you need. Heck, when you're really exhausted, it can be hard to even know where you parked your car! It's also okay not to know what you need. Simply asking the question helps us feel cared for. It validates the truth that our needs are important and worthy of being met. Still, you may gain clarity by asking the question more specifically to point you in the right direction, for example, "**What do I need . . .**"

- ☐ **To feel safe?** Do I need to get away and find some privacy?
- ☐ **To emotionally comfort myself?** Talk with a friend?
- ☐ **To physically soothe myself?** A warm bath or some exercise?
- ☐ **To encourage myself?** Read an inspiring book?
- ☐ **To protect myself?** Set a boundary with someone?
- ☐ **To provide for myself?** Get some rest or eat healthy food?
- ☐ **To take action?** Make a change?

> **The quintessential self-compassion question is "What do I need?"**

WHAT ARE "NEEDS" ANYWAY?

It's not always clear what we mean by "needs." Human beings may have an unlimited number of "wants," but our basic needs are relatively few. Needs are usually associated with survival. Some are *physical needs*, like food, clothing, shelter, exercise, and rest. On top of our physical needs, we have *mental and emotional needs*, such as the need for peace of mind, mental stimulation, or joy. Human beings are wired for connection, and we don't do well when our relationships are in trouble. Therefore, we also have *relational needs*, such as the need to be accepted, respected, valued, and loved.

If we feel burned out, chances are that many of our needs are not being met. We might not be getting enough sleep, we might not be eating well, perhaps we don't feel safe, or maybe we feel isolated and alone. When we're able to identify an unmet need and recognize it as a *universal* human need, we're more likely to feel entitled to address it even when the needs of others are in the forefront of our minds.

In contrast to needs, "wants" are desires that are not necessary for survival. For example, we might want a particular kind of entertainment or a type of food, but we can live without them. Wants tend to be personal rather than universal. Tallulah's desire for sparkly hair clips is an example of a want. Wants give us pleasure, and there's nothing wrong with pleasure, but if we confuse our needs and wants we'll have a harder time meeting our basic needs in the limited time we have available.

A helpful way to tell the difference between needs and wants is to put your hand over your heart when you ask the question "What do I need?" *Wants arise from the neck up, and needs come from the neck down.* We can have millions of wants, like we have millions of thoughts, but our needs are relatively simple and few. If you feel exhausted at the end of the day and put your hand over your heart and ask "What do I need now?" in a kind and sincere way, you're unlikely to say "An upgraded smartphone."

WHY DON'T WE ASK OURSELVES THE QUESTION?

It's not habitual for most of us to inquire about what we need. A common roadblock is feeling that we aren't worthy of getting our needs met. But like all human beings, you deserve to be happy and free from suffering. It's not selfish to provide for your needs—it's *necessary* as a responsible adult. Furthermore, if you make yourself miserable by disregarding your needs, people around you will also feel miserable. One thing you can always do for others is take good care of yourself.

Taking good care of yourself also benefits others.

But the roots of unworthiness go deep. At birth, nobody felt unworthy, but perhaps you didn't receive enough attention or affection in childhood and you concluded that you didn't deserve consideration and care. Cultural messages can also leave an unworthiness footprint. Sadly, mainstream cultures validate some identities and devalue others. Even if your parents were wholly supportive of who you are, when you step out the door your culture may still proclaim that somehow you're less worthy, and you internalize those messages. Winona, who was Navajo, had to struggle with this living in Albuquerque, where discrimination is still a fact of life, as it is in many places.

Our personalities are often shaped by feelings of unworthiness. For example, perfectionism (never good enough), crazy ambition (never successful enough), or excessive materialism (never enough stuff) can all be interpreted as efforts to convince ourselves or others that we're valuable and worthy. Unfortunately, the original wound of unworthiness gets obscured behind our elaborate efforts to prove our value.

Research shows that most people are more compassionate toward others than themselves. This is partly because society tells us it's selfish and self-indulgent to focus on our needs. For women this message is especially loud. Studies indicate that women have less self-compassion and more compassion for others than men, in part because they feel less entitled to meet their own needs. As mentioned in Chapter 3, this is not a matter of anatomy or gender identity (whether people are cisgendered, transgendered, or nonbinary) but of gender role socialization. Research has also shown that women allow themselves less free time than men and benefit less from it because they can't let go of worrying about other people.

Sometimes we don't focus on our own needs because we fear doing so will make us care less about others. Yet taking care of ourselves doesn't rob us of the capacity to care for others. Research has shown, in fact, that self-compassionate people are better able to take care of others, are more adept at compromise, and are more willing to seek a win–win solution by balancing their needs with those of others. If you don't meet your own needs, you'll find it very difficult to continue helping others as you become drained and depleted.

SELF-CARE AND SELF-COMPASSION

We hear the term *self-care* so much nowadays that it might make you roll your eyes. Through employer-mandated trainings and pop media advice, we've been inundated with exhortations to take a warm bath after a tough day at work, to go for a walk in healing nature, or to be sure to get a good night's sleep. Yoga classes? Sure, you can fit those in at around 4:00 a.m., before packing your kids' lunches, getting ready for work, looking over your notes for the first meeting of the day, and checking your email. No one ever tells you *how* you're supposed to fit self-care activities into your life. And it can be overwhelming to try, especially when you're burned out.

Self-care, as the term is commonly used, refers to behaviors we use to stay healthy and prevent suffering. Therefore, self-care falls under the umbrella of self-compassion. Self-care should be a guiding principle of everything we do, from choosing our friends to where we work, what we eat, and how we move our bodies. But the reality is, when we're at the end of our rope, we often don't have the time or energy.

Self-compassion is broader than self-care and includes how we relate to any moment of mental or emotional suffering. In fact, we can have compassion for the fact that we're too exhausted to practice basic self-care. You don't want to beat yourself up for not taking care of yourself, but you *do* want to ask yourself, "What do I need?" even if circumstances prevent you from taking the steps you'd ideally like to take. Self-compassion is an ongoing willingness to act in the interest of your own health and well-being, based on the understanding that your own needs are worthy of being met.

HOW THE THREE COMPONENTS OF SELF-COMPASSION CAN HELP

When we want to know what we need to ease burnout, the three components of self-compassion—self-kindness, common humanity, and mindfulness—can come to our aid by helping us cultivate *fulfilling, balanced authenticity.*

When we're kind to ourselves, we care about *fulfilling* our own needs. Kindness provides the warmth, validation, and support to affirm that our needs count. Even when we're burned out, kindness is the engine that drives us to take time for ourselves if we can, or at the very least to extend ourselves warmth and understanding when we can't. Meeting our needs becomes part of our approach to daily life, rather than a goal to be achieved sometime in the distant future.

Common humanity allows us to *balance* our needs with those of others. To be truly compassionate, our care must flow inward as well as outward. This allows us to step back, see the bigger picture, and figure out what's fair and workable for all. Focusing too much on our own needs could lead to a self-centered attitude that damages our relationships. Focusing too much on the needs of others could lead to a self-negating attitude that depletes us. Reminding ourselves that we're all humans, each with our own path to follow, helps us strike the right balance.

Mindfulness allows us to *authentically* answer the question "What do I need?" It turns our attention inward, facilitating introspection. When we lead an unexamined life, we sometimes go along with cultural programming that tells us we should put others' needs before our own. Or a consumeristic society that tells us what we should want—more money, more stuff, more praise—none of which brings lasting happiness. Research consistently shows that one of the primary benefits of self-compassion is greater authenticity. As we become less dependent on social approval for our sense of self-worth, we free ourselves to act according to our inner compass.

The following tool can help you meet your needs by tapping into the three components of self-compassion. You already learned variations of the self-compassion break aimed at tender acceptance (Chapter 6) and fierce protection (Chapter 14). This version is designed to evoke self-compassion when providing for our needs.

SELF-COMPASSION TOOL 16
Providing Self-Compassion Break

✦ Please think of an unmet need in your life related to burnout that you would like to address in this practice. Maybe you're exhausted and would like to get more rest, or your life has become a slog and you would benefit from more fun, or maybe you need time to reflect about possibly changing your career. Visualize the situation clearly in your mind.

✦ Allow yourself to feel whatever emotions are arising, such as grief, anger, fear, or despair. Make contact with the feelings as a physical sensation or energy.

✦ Now begin to shift your attention to see if you can name a physical, emotional, or relational human need that lies behind your unmet need, such as the need for health, rest, ease, safety, peace, joy, or connection.

✦ Next, sit up so that your body is alert. You're going to say a series of phrases designed to bring in the three components of self-compassion to help you take action to provide for yourself. Although words will be suggested, the goal is to find language that feels natural to you.

✦ The first phrase evokes mindfulness so you can become aware of what's true for you and recognize your authentic needs. Say to yourself with meaning, "This is what I authentically need to be healthy." Other options are "This is deeply meaningful to me" and "This is important to who I am."

✦ The second phrase is meant to help you remember common humanity so that you can include yourself in the circle of compassion and balance your needs with those of others. Try saying to yourself, "All humans have important needs, including me." Other options are "We all have needs that are worth being met" and "I will honor my needs as well as those of others."

✦ Now place both hands over your solar plexus (about two inches below your rib cage) and feel the warmth of your hands on your center.

✦ The third phrase expresses self-kindness by reminding you of your right to be fulfilled. Try saying to yourself something like "I deserve to be happy and free from suffering." Other options might be "I am committed to care for myself, no matter what, every day" and "I will do what is necessary to heal and thrive."

✦ If you're having difficulty finding the right words, imagine that someone you really cared about was feeling unfulfilled. What would you say to this person to help them respect their own needs and put in the time and effort necessary to feel better? Now, can you offer the same message to yourself?

✦ Finally, put one hand over your heart and leave the other hand over your solar plexus. The invitation is to combine the fierce energy of pursuing your needs with the tender energy of acceptance. Can you take action to be more fulfilled, while also realizing that you are already whole and complete exactly as you are? The desire to meet your needs doesn't come from a place of lack or deficiency, but from an abundant heart.

When Winona did this practice, she immediately thought of the need to reduce her high blood pressure. And underneath that, she realized she needed rest and more fun in her life. As she used mindfulness to become fully aware of how stressed she was, she realized how cut off she was from her body, which was crying for help. The next phrase, about common humanity—"All humans have important needs"—made her think of her daughter, who had needs that others did not. However, when Winona said, "My needs count too," and visualized herself along with Tallulah, she could feel the power of those words. Her own well-being was connected to her daughter's well-being. When she put her hands on her body and brought in self-kindness, saying, "I deserve to be happy and free from suffering," it was crystal clear to Winona that she needed to be healthy and strong not only to be a good mom but also to enjoy her life more.

In the final step—integrating fierce and tender self-compassion—she committed, then and there, to calling the respite center to see if they could take Tallulah for a week. Tallulah might feel a bit uncomfortable, but she would be okay. The moment she made this decision her whole body started to relax. Winona began to make the providing self-compassion break part of her regular routine. The old habits of self-sacrifice had started losing their grip, and eventually her blood pressure returned to normal levels.

In the next chapter, we build on meeting our needs and explore what brings *meaning* into our lives. Burnout is often a crisis of faith in ourselves, especially when we're in danger of abandoning our core principles and values. Healing includes sticking to your core values even when the circumstances of life are arrayed against you.

17

REDISCOVERING MEANING

What Are My Core Values?

A key feature of burnout is feeling disengaged from what's meaningful in life. Even when we're not collapsing from exhaustion or cranky from skipping meals, it may feel like something significant is missing at the end of the day. What happened to the satisfaction we got from a job well done? Where's the excitement we used to feel working on a team with our close colleagues? What happened to the sense of purpose, the fulfillment that came from knowing we were doing what we were meant to do, even though our days brought obstacles and dilemmas? Maybe we never realized how essential it is to live close to our values—to do the right thing, at the right time, with the right people—until it was gone.

Asking "What do I need?" starts the process of providing for ourselves when we're burned out. The next step in the process is to ask "What do I *value*?" or, more to the point, "What are my most important *core* values?" Needs and values go hand in hand. Meeting our needs allows us to survive, and living in accord with our core values makes life worth living.

When we're at the end of our rope, asking ourselves what we value in life may seem like an unaffordable luxury. But connecting with our core values is not a luxury; it's a necessity. Our core values provide a natural source of strength and vitality. Cutting ourselves off from this inner wellspring is partly what makes us feel so drained and empty.

Jason, a talkative young cop with a fondness for telling stories, hasn't had much to say for the past few months. He's been horrified by the attention that police brutality has been getting in the news. He's also been weighed down by the arguments it has caused among fellow cops in his own precinct, most of whom were not racist and resented being portrayed as such given the fact that they put their lives on the line every day.

But Jason wasn't so sure about his partner and mentor, Stan. When they pull a car over for a traffic violation, he notices that Stan asks more questions of Black drivers than White ones. He's also more aggressive with Black drivers, even though he doesn't seem to realize what he's doing. Should Jason say something to Stan, or would that be disloyal? Should he stay silent, or would that be tacitly supporting injustice?

This wasn't how it was supposed to be. Jason's father and uncle were retired cops who had been at Ground Zero on 9/11. They taught him about three essentials in police work: loyalty, justice, and duty to protect. These values played an important role in Jason's lifelong dream of joining the police force, and it made him extremely uncomfortable to operate out of alignment with these values.

Policing is dangerous and stressful enough. The fact that he was losing trust in his partner made it doubly stressful. One morning while shaving, Jason sees the same sunken eyes he sometimes noticed on his dad's face just before he retired at age sixty. Jason is only twenty-six. He becomes flooded with shame as he imagines telling his father that he can't hack it. He feels like a failure.

Moral Injury

When our actions are at odds with our moral values, we can experience moral injury. *Moral injury* refers to the anguish—grief, shame, anger, disgust—that results when we witness or engage in behaviors that violate our own deeply held moral values. It occurs when we know the right thing to do, but circumstances make it impossible to pursue the right course of action. Moral injury is often traumatic and can have serious consequences, including posttraumatic stress, depression, substance abuse, and self-harm. It occurs not only in the military and police force but also among health care professionals or in fields like education, when constraints such as paperwork or budget concerns prevent people from providing needed services. Research suggests that the stress of moral injury can contribute to burnout.

RECONNECTING WITH OUR VALUES

Research shows that, like Jason, we're more likely to criticize and blame ourselves when our actions at work are at odds with our personal and moral values, resulting in moral injury (see the box on the preceding page). Fortunately, self-compassion can help when facing moral injury and softens its impact. How does it work? Instead of judging and shaming ourselves for being out of sync with our values, we're kind and understanding. We realize it's part of being human and are more able to keep things in perspective. But being self-compassionate when we're burned out also means doing what we can to get back on track and live with integrity.

Living in alignment with our values not only reduces stress but provides big benefits. Research shows that people whose lives are infused with meaning feel more contentment, satisfaction, happiness, and joy; they have better relationships and physical health; they even sleep better. Studies also show that living in accord with our values helps us feel authentic—at home in our own skin and connected to the wider world. When we lose touch with our core values somewhere along the road to burnout, the self-compassionate thing to do is to name them and reclaim them.

KNOWING YOUR CORE VALUES

Core values have become a popular subject in recent years, especially in the fields of business, education, and psychology. For example, core values are central to the acceptance and commitment therapy (ACT) model of psychotherapy that informs much of this chapter. Core values can be defined as the beliefs, principles, and ideals that define our identity and guide our choices. They are our *north star*—helping us chart the course of our lives.

A huge number of lists of core values is available online—one Google search for "core values list" yielded over a billion results! If you're not sure what your core values are, exploring a list and looking for what resonates is one way to start. Listed on the next page you'll find sixty core values, drawn from various sources and listed in no particular order, to give you an idea of what we mean. At the end of this chapter you'll have a chance to explore your own core values in the context of self-compassion.

Sample Core Values

1. Adventure
2. Humor
3. Peace
4. Beauty
5. Curiosity
6. Logic
7. Humility
8. Loyalty
9. Tolerance
10. Love
11. Compassion
12. Prosperity
13. Intuition
14. Learning
15. Spirituality
16. Cooperation
17. Achievement
18. Kindness
19. Equality
20. Nature
21. Balance
22. Contribution
23. Duty
24. Integrity
25. Harmony
26. Creativity
27. Forgiveness
28. Friendliness
29. Fame
30. Service
31. Tradition
32. Generosity
33. Popularity
34. Responsibility
35. Fun
36. Growth
37. Independence
38. Openness
39. Productivity
40. Health
41. Courage
42. Wisdom
43. Competence
44. Self-awareness
45. Patriotism
46. Honor
47. Gratitude
48. Self-control
49. Enjoyment
50. Honesty
51. Power
52. Logic
53. Safety
54. Respect
55. Self-care
56. Goodness
57. Authenticity
58. Family
59. Ethics
60. Intelligence

CORE VALUES VERSUS SOCIAL NORMS

Sometimes the values that seem to be guiding us are actually social norms that we've been taught to follow. Social norms are rules of acceptable behavior in society. Values are beliefs about what is important, which may or may not overlap with social norms. For example, "going to school" is a norm, and "growth and learning" would be a value. "Family loyalty" could be *both* a social norm and a value. Sometimes social norms and values conflict. Colin Kaepernick, an American football player who knelt during the playing of the national anthem, broke the social norm of standing during the anthem. The ensuing controversy centered on whether people felt his act violated the core value of patriotism or supported the core value of racial justice. If you have a core value in mind and you're wondering if it's really a social norm, ask yourself if you feel energized by following it. If the answer is yes, it's probably a core value. If it depletes your energy, it's probably a social norm.

Core values energize us; social norms often deplete us. You may have started doing your job because you felt you "should" do that type of work and your heart was never in it. In that case you might have been motivated by a social norm rather than a core value. There's no shame in that, but it may be contributing to your feelings of burnout. If you're going to recover your vitality, it's important to understand what really matters to you. You need to know what is authentically your own. Living in accord with our authentic core values brings out the best in us. As Maya Angelou wrote, "If you are always trying to be normal you will never know how amazing you can be."

GOALS VERSUS CORE VALUES

It's difficult to focus on anything but goals when we're under pressure from so many demands: What do I need to get done today? How can I make this quota or meet that deadline? Why does my to-do list always get longer instead of shorter? Out of necessity, we often pay most of our attention to getting things done without pausing to consider *why* we're doing what we're doing. We're only looking for the finish line.

To stay on a course that has meaning for us, it's helpful to make sure we can distinguish our core values from our goals. Goals are specific results that we can achieve through our actions, whereas core values are what motivate and guide our actions. For example, your core value might be to live a life of service to humanity, and a goal might be to get an advanced degree so that you can acquire the skills and social capital to serve more effectively. After you get your degree, you can continue in the direction of your north star—service to humanity. In other words, goals can be achieved; core values guide us *up to* and *after* achieving our goals.

Goals are destinations; core values are directions.

Goals are also something we *do*; core values are something we *are*. Our core values are the axis around which our lives revolve. When people gather at a funeral, the most consistent theme of the eulogy is usually the deceased's core values. For example, maybe the deceased always fought for the underdog (core value: social justice) or was irrepressible in telling the truth (core value: honesty). As we age, we may identify as a child, an adult, or an older person, but our core values are who we *really* are.

Interestingly, we don't *choose* our core values. If we did, they would probably be infiltrated by social norms. Core values are *discovered*. Our lived experienced tells us what's truly meaningful to us. But once we've discovered our core values, we need to remind ourselves about them so we don't get lost. And if we're lost, core values can show us the way home.

RETURNING HOME

Exploring our core values yields all sorts of surprises. When we're burned out, some people discover that the career that's draining them doesn't reflect their values at all and that they were pushed into that line of work by well-meaning parents, teachers, or friends. Others find that their work used to align with their values but no longer does. And sometimes we find that what we used to value is not so meaningful anymore.

Where are *you* right now? Do any of these people seem familiar?

- Reggie went into medicine because everyone in his family was a doctor, but he realizes a core value is *creativity* and his real love in life is music.

- Wanda went into the hospitality industry because a core value for her is *social connection*, but now she's burned out because, as a hotel manager, her encounters with people are mostly about managing complaints.

- Kumiko is a successful tech executive who got where she was through developing new products. Right now, she's stuck managing people and answering to the board of directors. Her core value of *innovation* is in jeopardy.

- Vlad is a civil litigation lawyer who used to value *money and power*, but now that he has kids his career doesn't fit his value of *quality time with family*.

When we find that our work isn't aligned with our core values, it may be time to make a change. However, we don't need to change *everything* in our lives. Small changes that reflect our core values can lift us up even when big changes aren't possible. In the examples given on the previous page, Reggie started having R&B music piped into his medical suite. Kumiko started a weekly dinner brainstorming with friends who were working on IT projects of their own. Just these small acts of commitment to their core values made a big difference to them and can do the same for you.

The following tool will help you reconnect with your core values. Finding your true north will not fix burnout once and for all, but it will help guide you on the path to recovery. In this exercise, you'll start bringing awareness to what matters most in your life—your core values—and learn to be compassionate with yourself when you *can't* live in accord with your values.

SELF-COMPASSION TOOL 17
Discovering Your Core Values

✦ Imagine that you're in your elderly years, or at least ten to twenty years older than you are now. You're sitting in a lovely garden as you contemplate your life. Looking back, you feel a deep sense of satisfaction, joy, and contentment. Even though life hasn't always been easy, you managed to stay true to yourself to the best of your ability. Which core values did you live by that gave your life meaning? (If you like, please see the core values list on page 151 for suggestions.) Write down one or more core values.

✦ Now write down any ways you feel you are *not living in accord with your core values*, or ways that your life feels out of balance with your values. For example, perhaps you value peace but are continually being drawn into conflicts at work, or perhaps you value fun but find you don't have time to laugh or play anymore.

✦ Might any of these areas of imbalance be contributing to your feelings of burnout, and if so, how?

✦ There are often obstacles that prevent us from living in accord with our core values. Some of these may be *external obstacles*, like not having enough money or having too many family responsibilities. If you have any such obstacles, please note them.

✦ There may also be some *internal obstacles* getting in the way of your living in accord with your core values. For instance, you might not feel worthy of following your dreams, perhaps you're uncomfortable speaking up, or you doubt yourself. Please write down any internal obstacles you might have.

✦ Now consider whether self-compassion could help you *live in accord with your core values*. For example, could it help you feel safe and confident enough to take new actions, risk rejection, or stop doing things that are a waste of your time? Or might self-compassion encourage you to rest when you're tired, because you *deserve* to take time out to rest, or might a bit of fierce self-compassion motivate you to find a different job?

✦ If there are *insurmountable obstacles* to living in accord with your core values—obligations that you just can't avoid, for instance—can you give yourself compassion for your current situation? Can you offer yourself words of kindness and understanding as you might to a good friend? Or can you encourage yourself to persevere despite the odds and not abandon your core values?

✦ Finally, is there any creative way you can bring your values into your life, even if their expression is incomplete? For instance, maybe a core value is spending time in nature, yet you work in an office all day. Can you fill your office with plants or commit to taking a walk in the woods every weekend? Are there small things you can do to live more in alignment with your values? If so, please write these down too.

When Jason did this exercise, he had no trouble visualizing himself as an older person looking back on his life. His core values were still the same—loyalty, justice, and the duty to protect. However, he felt a weight in his stomach when he realized the way his partner was treating people wasn't in line with his value of justice. And he couldn't simply separate his partner's actions from his own; they worked as a team. The moral injury he was experiencing was becoming more painful with each passing day. The external obstacle that Jason was able to identify was the prevailing culture and the larger historical context of racism that created more suspicion of Black people. But Jason's main internal obstacle was his strong wish for recognition and approval from Stan, which kept him from speaking up.

At first Jason felt ashamed of being a coward, but he gave himself compassion for not calling Stan out. It was only natural that he wanted to maintain a good relationship with his partner. And loyalty was also one of his core values. He resolved to speak with Stan privately and respectfully in a way that (hopefully) strengthened their relationship rather than pulling them apart. He also decided to join an online community of police officers in his state committed to racial equity in policing, as a small step in the right direction.

Overall, this exploration of core values left Jason feeling sadder but wiser. He said it "helped me grow up." He realized that the police force was made up of people like him, imperfect human beings, and that his personal values might sometimes be at odds with those of others. Jason felt confident that no matter what happened—even if he had to request a different partner—he would be okay.

Self-compassion is personal, so discovering your unique, authentic core values is key to recovering from burnout. Finding your north star and remaining true to it while feeling exhausted and hollow is no easy task, however. It helps to have a coach who keeps you on track and reminds you of who you are. Fortunately, each of us has such a person available 24/7. The next chapter will show you how to engage your inner coach to motivate you to make change in your life and realize your full potential.

18

BECOMING A WISE INNER COACH

Self-Compassionate Motivation

Once we attend to that big hole where our meaning and purpose in life resided before we got so wrung out, we might feel an itch to get moving again. But it can be hard to take the first step . . . and the second . . . and the third.

Maybe you want to change the work you do in the world, but you're not sure how. Doubts about your work can lead to self-doubt, and before you know it, that old familiar voice of self-criticism is reverberating in your head: "Why can't you just figure this out?" "Stop feeling sorry for yourself and grow up!"

At times like these it helps to have a mentor and supportive coach. You need to hear that you'll get there, that you're up to the challenge even if you feel anything but, and that you can make meaningful change as long as you're patient and persistent. You need constructive criticism, not admonishment. Think Ted Lasso or Obi-Wan Kenobi. Imagine the best boss or teacher you ever had or your go-to friend, the one who gives it to you straight but never at the high price of tearing you down. Old habits die hard, however, and we're more used to spurring ourselves forward with insult and intimidation. We don't realize that self-compassion is more effective at pulling us out of the tar pit.

> **Self-compassion is a better motivator than self-criticism because it comes from love and not fear.**

Ellie is a scriptwriter for a reality TV show who is at the end of her rope, and the longer she stays at her job, the more it seems to crush the life out of her. The hours are long—she works twelve- to fourteen-hour shifts, six days a week—and she doesn't get any writing credit (viewers assume all the dialogue is spontaneous). But the income is steady, and she's been able to save some money. The problem is, for all its material benefits, this show is not what she wanted to do—even a little. Putting words designed to promote infighting and drama into the mouths of contestants is not terribly interesting or challenging, and over time Ellie has started feeling depressed. She feels like a fraud for writing such schlock and knows she's capable of far better work. Hadn't she won a significant literary prize in college? Ellie dreams of writing a great screenplay based on a story idea she's been toying with for years. If she could get enough written to interest a producer, maybe she could quit her current job and work on the screenplay full time.

Ellie tries to push herself using shame and ridicule. "You can't keep being a second-rate hack forever. If you want to be a real writer, you need to draft at least ten pages a week. You don't want to be a dried-up loser, do you?" But Ellie struggles to write even half a paragraph. She's so tired at the end of the day she can't bear the thought of opening her laptop and working a moment longer. So she ramps up the self-criticism, afraid that if she lets herself off the hook she'll be stuck in reality show hell forever.

BUT WON'T YOU GET SOFT?

Like Ellie, many people resist self-compassion because they're afraid it will make them lose their drive. They think self-compassion just means going easy on yourself. It doesn't. Self-compassion focuses on the alleviation of suffering. Sure, sometimes that means taking a break or scaling back—especially when you're exhausted and overextended. But if at some point this prevents you from moving forward to follow your dreams, you're actually causing suffering, not alleviating it.

When we care about ourselves, we don't do this. The tender, accepting side of self-compassion allows us to see our behavior clearly without judgment, so we can recognize when our self-care is veering dangerously close to self-indulgence. The fierce, action-oriented side of self-compassion then kicks into gear, driving us to expend the effort needed to help ourselves thrive and be happy.

Inspiration Rather than Insults

When we call ourselves nasty names to try to motivate ourselves, as Ellie does when she stares at a blank page, we're following the dog-eared playbook of bad coaches everywhere. These hard-liners believe that demeaning their players is the only way to propel them to a new level of excellence. That's because they've seen it work, at least temporarily. But being screamed at doesn't motivate players to improve in the long run, if at all; it just gives them a shot of adrenaline so they can escape the coach's now-terrifying wrath.

Harsh criticism is an ineffective coaching technique, whether it's aimed outward or inward. It robs us of the energy and self-confidence we need to get where we really want to go. It also makes it harder for us to learn from our mistakes: shame hollows out our sense of self to the point that there's no one left to see what went wrong or where to go next.

Being compassionate toward ourselves when we fail leaves us better able to learn from our setbacks. Remember the study done with NCAA athletes discussed in Chapter 12? Players trained to use warm and constructive self-feedback about mistakes in games or training routines were more able to take in the information and use it. They improved their athletic performance as a result. Other studies show that self-compassionate people tend to have a growth mindset rather than a fixed mindset. Carol Dweck, a well-known research psychologist who studies learning, proposes that people with a fixed mindset who feel their abilities are set in stone are more likely to see failure as a sign of being incompetent or inadequate. Those with a growth mindset

> **Self-compassion fosters a growth mindset and allows us to learn from our mistakes.**

who believe their abilities can be improved tend to see failure as a learning opportunity. That's partly why teaching athletes self-compassion was so effective—it engendered a growth mindset. It moved players away from the default auto-response of "I failed, so I must be a failure" to "What can I learn from this?"

This is a powerful pivot. Mark Williamson, the director of the UK's Action for Happiness Organization, came up with a novel way of making this shift. He used to reflexively beat himself up for every misstep, calling himself a f——ing idiot without thought. Now that he's learned about self-compassion he uses a simple acronym to remind himself of what's needed instead: "Friendly, Useful, Calm, Kind." That's the definition of a good coach in four simple words.

WHERE DO YOU NEED GUIDANCE?

A key goal of those in the coaching profession is to find out what clients are trying to do and then help them do it. The same can be said of good therapists. When we counsel people who are struggling, our goal is to help them get where they want to go. People consult coaches and counselors for a variety of reasons, such as to get a business started, make career changes, improve their marital communication, or learn a new skill.

Are there aspects of your life related to burnout that you would like guidance on?

❑ Changing careers?

❑ Making your work resonate more with your values?

❑ Working fewer hours?

❑ Creating a better work–life balance?

❑ Dealing with challenging relationships?

❑ Finding time for more self-care?

❑ Learning to say no?

When we're so burned out that we just want to crawl into bed and pull the covers over our head, motivating ourselves to make a life change may seem like an impossibly tall order. Fortunately, the wisdom and compassion that reside in all of us can serve as a supportive inner coach, helping us along the way. We can take a good, hard look at the circumstances that got us into this mess and provide constructive feedback on how to get out of it. We can also take responsibility for our contributions to the situation and be supportive and understanding as we learn to do things differently.

MOTIVATING OURSELVES USING THE THREE COMPONENTS OF SELF-COMPASSION

The desire to alleviate our suffering drives us to make changes in our lives not because we're inadequate as we are, but because we care about ourselves

and want to be happy. When we use fierce self-compassion for motivation, we experience *encouraging, wise vision*.

Kindness

The kindness component of self-compassion expresses itself as **encouragement** when you're burned out. Encouragement doesn't mean lying to yourself that everything's great even when it isn't. Such lies ring hollow, backfire, and just make you feel worse. Kindness acknowledges our problems and limitations, but it does so with warmth and understanding. It's not interested in tearing us down, but in building us up. It gently pushes us to do whatever we can to improve our situation, trusting that we will catch ourselves if we fall. It establishes the sense of safety we need to take risks, inspiring us to follow our dreams of growth and discovery. It also provides grit and determination in the face of obstacles, so that when we get knocked down we can pick ourselves up and try again.

Common Humanity

Our sense of our common humanity takes shape as **wisdom** when we try to motivate change. We recognize that being human means making mistakes, getting it wrong, failing, and getting stuck. When we forget our humanity, we unconsciously believe that we *shouldn't* struggle and that there's something wrong with us when we do. We get so overwhelmed by the feelings of shame and self-blame that go along with failure that we can't see clearly, which inhibits our ability to learn and grow.

It's helpful here to distinguish between harsh judgment and discriminating wisdom. Harsh judgment involves a narrow, rigid labeling of ourselves as "good" or "bad." Discriminating wisdom identifies what's working and what isn't, what's healthy or harmful, but does so in full knowledge of the complex, dynamic factors influencing the situation. We can judge our performances or achievements as good or bad without taking things personally. Just because I failed doesn't mean that I am somehow "a failure." By framing our experience in the larger context of what it means to be human, we gain insight and knowledge that helps us move forward.

Mindfulness

Mindfulness provides focus and **vision** when we're trying to recover from burnout. Exhaustion makes us feel like our head is in a fog. But we need to be aware of what's happening, how we got there, and where we're going if we're ever going to improve our lives. When we stop resisting the reality of burnout, we're better able to gain the clarity and perspective needed to chart a new path. When we pay attention to our present-moment experience, we can connect the dots to envision how things might unfold in the future. Mindfulness is like shining a bright light that allows us to see where we're going. It helps us stick to our goal of healing and recovery without getting distracted by those voices in our head telling us we aren't capable of changing.

Self-compassion provides the encouraging, wise vision that has always been available to you but has been in hiding during burnout. Here is a tool that can help you stay in touch with these self-compassionate qualities when you're trying to motivate yourself to learn and grow in a meaningful way.

SELF-COMPASSION TOOL 18
Motivating Self-Compassion Break

✦ Please think about a goal you'd like to reach that could help reduce your feelings of burnout. Maybe you'd like to get a new job or negotiate more support or reduced work hours from your boss, or take better care of your body by exercising more, or improve your communication with a family member you care for.

✦ What feelings arise when you think about trying to reach this goal—frustration, disappointment, fear, confusion, or perhaps shame? Make contact with the emotions as physical sensations in your body.

✦ Make sure your posture is upright and you aren't slumping. Roll your shoulders back.

✦ Here are a few phrases that you can say silently to yourself, designed to bring in the three components of self-compassion so that you can try to motivate yourself to achieve your goal with encouragement and support. As always, the aim is to find language that makes sense to you and feels natural.

✦ The first phrase brings in mindfulness, so that you have a clear vision of what you'd like to achieve and the benefits that reaching the goal would have for you. Try saying to yourself slowly and with conviction, "This is what I want for myself." Other options are "This goal is important to me" and "This would bring me happiness."

✦ The second phrase calls on the wisdom of common humanity. We remember that everyone gets stuck, fails, and makes mistakes, but we learn from our experience. Try saying to yourself, "Learning from failure is part of being human." Other options include "We usually get it wrong before we get it right" and "Growth is usually slow and messy."

✦ Now offer yourself a supportive gesture, such as putting one hand on the opposite shoulder or doing a small fist pump to signal encouragement.

✦ Imagine that inside of you there is a wise, supportive, effective coach who has some words of encouragement for you. What would this kind coach say? "I believe in you," I will support you," or "Just try your best and see what happens."

✦ Is there any constructive criticism or useful feedback your inner coach would offer?

✦ If you're having difficulty finding the right words, imagine that you were mentoring someone who had a similar goal and you wanted to support them in achieving their aims. What would you say? What would your tone of voice be like? Is there any constructive criticism you would offer? Now, can you offer the same message to yourself?

✦ Finally, allow the fierce energy of encouraging, wise vision to combine with the tender energy of unconditional self-acceptance. We want to reach our goals not because we're inadequate as we are, but because we want to alleviate our suffering. We can try our best to achieve our objectives, but the bottom line is that it's okay if we don't. We are loved and lovable exactly as we are right now.

Doing this practice was like a shot in the arm for Ellie. She knew what she wanted to do, but it was too much to write her screenplay while working on the reality show full-time. She had saved enough money to live for about six months, however, so theoretically she could take a hiatus from the show for the rest of the season and devote herself to writing full-time. This thought excited her but also terrified her. It felt like jumping off a cliff.

First, she used mindfulness to gain perspective and said calmly, "This is my vision for myself." She knew that it was possible for her, especially since she could draw on her savings. She just had to focus and keep her eye on the prize.

Tapping into the wisdom of common humanity is really what shifted things, however. She realized she was unconsciously falling into the trap of self-sabotage. Her current job gave her an excuse for not writing the screenplay. She wanted so badly to be a good writer that she didn't dare put herself out there in case she wasn't. But the realization that she would never learn the craft of screenwriting without giving it her full effort got her past her fear of failure.

She put her left hand on her heart to comfort herself for how afraid she was and used the right hand to do a little fist pump. It felt a bit hokey and contrived, but oddly comforting.

She started giving herself a little pep talk, just like the professor who had helped her earn that literary prize. "Hey, Ellie. I know it's scary, but taking this leap is the only way you're ever going to become the writer you've dreamed of being. Yes, your screenplay might get rejected at first. That's the way it works. Hopefully you'll get some good feedback so you can improve your work. Your story idea is a good one, and you have natural talent. Now you just have to hone your craft."

When Ellie said this, she heard a scared little voice whisper, "But what if I don't have the talent? What if I don't have what it takes?" Bringing in tender self-compassion really helped at this point. She gave herself a hug and said, "You know, Ellie, it's okay if you never make it as a screenwriter. I love you whether you're talented or not! I want you to try because I believe in you and want you to make your best effort. But if it doesn't work out, I won't love you any less." This unconditional reassurance gave Ellie a tremendous feeling of safety. And also freedom. She would just try her best and see what happened. It might even be fun!

Motivating ourselves with compassion is like giving plants water and fertilizer—it helps us grow and thrive. This continual encouragement cultivates a mindset of goodwill and benevolence. In traditional Buddhist meditation practice, the practice of goodwill is referred to as *loving-kindness practice*. In the next chapter, you'll learn how to strengthen the muscles of loving-kindness and to speak to yourself in a warm, supportive way throughout the day. This warmth can help counter the debilitating effects of burnout.

GOODWILL, NOT GOOD FEELINGS

Cultivating Loving-Kindness

Sometimes we're told that to lighten the dark cloud of burnout we need to think positively. Pop psychology promises that our dreams of feeling better will come true if we just look in the mirror and repeat a few words of positive affirmation, like "Every day in every way I am getting stronger and stronger." NOT! In your burned-out state, would you believe such baloney? Arjun certainly wouldn't.

Arjun is a veteran respiratory therapist. He's in good physical shape, but mentally and emotionally he's not doing so well. Ever since COVID he's been stretched to his limit, not just by the extra hours he's had to work but by the emotional toll wreaked by the pandemic. So many people's lives he watched slip away, despite his best efforts to keep oxygen flowing into their lungs. So many long COVID sufferers with scarred lungs or recurrent shortness of breath. And despite all the vaccines, COVID seems like it's here to stay.

Arjun tries to give his patients hope as he looks into their pleading eyes. He smiles and acts as if everything will be fine, even though he knows it might not be. This fake cheerfulness seems to help some people, but it isn't working for him. He feels oddly detached from his patients, as if he's watching them from behind a glass wall. He doesn't feel capable of doing his job anymore. He's exhausted yet can't sleep at night. In other words, he's burned out, big time. Arjun used to be a happy and optimistic guy. He wants to find a way back to his pre-COVID self but can't seem to figure out how to get there.

Pretending we're happy does not make it so. Telling ourselves that we feel a particular way when we don't is like being gaslighted—and by the person we should be able to trust the most, ourselves. "I'm okay, you're okay" may sound like an acknowledgment of our common humanity, except it lacks self-compassion if it's based on a lie. *No one who is burned out is okay.*

Positive affirmations say "I'm okay, you're okay."

Self-compassion says "I'm not okay, you're not okay . . . but that's okay!"

We don't want to pretend things are going swimmingly when we feel like we're drowning. Trying to change reality only postpones the healing process. We can't change the reality of this moment—regardless of which spells, magic wands, and rabbits we pull out of a hat. And yet that doesn't mean we should be glum about it all either.

Research shows that self-compassionate people tend to be more hopeful and optimistic than those who are cold to themselves. That's because when we have compassion for our struggles in the present, we generate goodwill toward ourselves that makes the future appear brighter.

CULTIVATING LOVING-KINDNESS

There is a form of goodwill training that has existed for centuries called *loving-kindness meditation*, in which a series of phrases is repeated to cultivate friendliness toward ourselves and others. It's not a million miles from the practice of positive affirmations, but instead of saying "I am [fill in the blank]" as a way to manifest the desired state, which potentially sets up an argument with the truth, we say "May I [fill in the blank]" to express our positive intentions for ourselves. Traditional phrases include:

May I be safe.

May I be happy.

May I be healthy.

May I live with ease.

These phrases are like wishes or blessings. We repeat loving-kindness phrases to cultivate benevolent intentions rather than particular mood states.

Loving-kindness focuses on the *wish* for health and well-being. We acknowledge how terrible we feel, but also our heart's desire to feel better. Loving-kindness phrases like "May I be happy" are meant to evoke goodwill, not good feelings.

Loving-kindness practice may seem counterintuitive. It's another iteration of the paradox of self-compassion (see Chapter 9): we give ourselves compassion not to feel better but because we feel bad. If we practice loving-kindness with an expectation of feeling better, we're resisting reality, and what we resist persists or grows stronger. Instead, we wish ourselves well even though we're hurting, and this benevolence helps us cope with our pain and eventually move on from it.

THE DIFFERENCE BETWEEN LOVING-KINDNESS AND SELF-COMPASSION

Loving-kindness and self-compassion are two sides of the same coin. Both are expressions of warmth and care, but self-compassion specifically refers to caring in the midst of suffering (*passion* in Latin means "suffering"). Loving-kindness refers to goodwill more generally and isn't necessarily focused on suffering. It includes positive emotions like joy and happiness and looks to the future as well as the present. A Burmese monk once put it this way: "When the sunshine of loving-kindness meets the tears of suffering, the rainbow of compassion appears."

But warmth is warmth: loving-kindness and compassion go hand in hand. Research shows that practicing traditional loving-kindness meditation increases self-compassion and that practicing self-compassion increases joy and happiness. This is good news, because sometimes we don't want to focus on our suffering. When we're burned out, we may need a break from our trouble and strife. By cultivating loving-kindness, we can elevate our mood without denying our pain. It's like sunbathing on the beach (without the need for sunscreen!).

HOW DOES LOVING-KINDNESS WORK?

Think of loving-kindness practice as a workout at the gym for our heart muscles, which have gotten atrophied through the experience of burnout. The stress of our work causes us to pull away from life and go into a shell. The feelings of disconnection and apathy that are part of burnout are indicators that our heart has shut down to protect itself. By setting our *intention* to cultivate goodwill, even if we aren't fully feeling it, we can start to reverse things.

There is a touching Hasidic tale that illustrates how loving-kindness practice works. A disciple asks his rebbe, "Why does Torah tell us to 'place these words upon your hearts'? Why does it not tell us to place these holy words in our hearts?" The rebbe answers, "It is because as we are, our hearts are closed, and we cannot place the holy words in our hearts. So we place them on top of our hearts. And there they stay until, one day, the heart breaks and the words fall in."

Our intentions shape us, like the conductor in a locomotive pulling a train that carries our thoughts in one car, our emotions in another car, and our behaviors in a third. If we don't set our intention to recover from burnout, we can get dragged along by a runaway train with no conductor: we work harder and longer, deny ourselves the rest and nutrition we need, and out of sheer frustration start lashing out at ourselves and others. We are pulled by forces that feel beyond our control.

But you can install goodwill as your conductor, bringing along with it healthier thoughts, emotions, and behaviors. When you say to yourself, "I wish you well," you begin to believe that you are worthy of being well. This helps you feel safe and loved. You may then start to act in ways that will help counter burnout, such as drawing boundaries or meeting your needs. But nothing is going to change unless you set your intention to heal.

Because charting a new course takes effort, and effort is in short supply when you're burned out, loving-kindness should be as easy as possible. That's why it helps to find simple goodwill phrases that you can call up throughout the day. And whether or not you actually remember to say the words, *simply setting the intention to offer yourself words of kindness is a big step forward.* It's okay to just go through the motions if that's all you can manage. This is not a command performance.

When we repeat loving-kindness phrases even if we're not feeling them, not only are we setting our intentions

> **Whether or not you actually feel kind and loving, repeating loving-kindness phrases sets your intention to heal.**

in the right direction, we're also countering old habits. In other words, we're not doing what we're usually doing—focusing on how horrible things are. Being briefly interrupted from rumination is a break from the downward spiral of negativity we often get trapped by, and any break is useful for countering burnout.

HOW TO CRAFT LOVING-KINDNESS PHRASES

The phrases we choose for loving-kindness practice should be deeply meaningful to us and get at the heart of the answer to the kindest question of all: "What do I need?" Authenticity is key. If we use phrases that don't reflect what really matters to us, uttering them will feel as empty as saying "Have a good day!" at the end of a phone call.

It's helpful to settle on a few phrases you can easily memorize and repeat, but they need not be set in stone. You can change your phrases whenever you choose. The following tool will help you find phrases that allow your heart to rest.

Suggestions for Finding Meaningful Loving-Kindness Phrases

✦ Choose phrases that are not only authentic but also simple, clear, and kind.

✦ Think of finding loving-kindness phrases as writing poetry, calling in the attitude of loving-kindness using evocative words that are specifically meaningful to you.

✦ Be general rather than specific. Rather than "May I get a new job that has fewer working hours," try broader phrases like "May I live with ease."

✦ Choose phrases that feel like slipping into a warm bath or sunbathing on a beach. Like the water or sun, the phrases do all the work, and all you need to do is show up. *A good loving-kindness phrase is one that allows the heart to rest.*

✦ Choose phrases that don't cause any argument in your head. For instance, instead of "May I be free from stress," choose something more realistic, such as "May I have moments of peace every day."

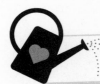

SELF-COMPASSION TOOL 19
Finding Loving-Kindness Phrases

The purpose of this practice is to find a few loving-kindness phrases that are powerful and personally meaningful. These phrases can be repeated silently in meditation, spoken aloud in the shower, written on sticky notes, or whispered as you walk to work. They can be used anywhere at any time, as a reminder that you care about yourself. Once memorized, the phrases may also arise spontaneously when needed in daily life to comfort, support, or encourage you.

Try to say the phrases slowly and with warmth. The *tone* with which you say the phrases matters a great deal. It's like talking to an infant or a beloved pet who responds to *how* you speak more than *what* you say. Rushing—as so many burned-out people are used to doing—is unnecessary and may create a sense of tension.

What Do I Need?

✦ To start, please put a hand over your heart or elsewhere and feel your body breathe gently. Then take a moment and allow your heart to open gently—to become receptive—the way a flower opens in the warm sun.

✦ Focus on your feelings of burnout. Now ask yourself, "What do I need? What do I truly need?" and allow the answer to arise naturally within you: let the answer be a *universal* human need that is not being met, such as the need to be "valued," "healthy," "peaceful," "connected," or "safe." What do you feel is missing as you experience the stress and depletion of burnout?

✦ Please write down what arises for you.

✦ The words you discovered can be used just as they are—for example, "I need support" or "I need rest"—or you can rewrite your needs as wishes for yourself, such as:

- "May I have stability."
- "May I experience peace."
- "May I be courageous."
- "May I trust in myself."
- "May I let go of fear."

What Do I Need to *Hear*?

✦ Now consider a second question: "What do I need to hear from others? What words do I long to hear because, as a person suffering burnout, I really need to hear words like this?" Open the door of your heart and wait for words to come. Ask yourself, "If I could, what words would I like to have whispered into my ear every day—both now, while feeling the way I do, and after emerging from burnout—for the rest of my life?" Words that might make you say, "Oh, thank you, thank you" every time you hear them. Allow yourself to be vulnerable and open to this possibility, with courage.

✦ Write down what you hear.

✦ Once again, the words you wrote down can be used just as they are, or you can rewrite them as wishes for yourself. Often words that we would like to hear from others reflect qualities we would like to actualize in ourselves, and we can write phrases that express this wish. For example:

- "I love you" can become the wish "May I know that I am lovable."
- "I'll support you and help you" can become the wish "May I take good care of myself."
- "You're a good person" can become the wish "May I know that I deserve compassion."
- "You're important to me" can become the wish "May I know that I matter."

✦ Look through what you've written and pick one or two phrases that really resonate for you. Take a moment to memorize these words or phrases.

✦ Now try them out to see how they land inside you. Begin saying your phrases over and over to yourself, slowly and gently, as if whispering them into the ear of a loved one. Try to hear the words from the inside, allowing them to resonate within you, to take up space, to fill your being.

✦ Finally, gently release the phrases, allowing this practice to be just as it was and letting yourself be just as you are.

In his search for meaningful loving-kindness phrases, Arjun realized that what he really needed was to feel less overwhelmed by death and chronic debilitation. So he wrote down that he needed "peace" and "joy." He then turned these into wishes: "May I experience peace and joy." But that felt like too tall an order, so he modified the phrase to "May I live in peace and joy as often as possible."

When he considered what he wanted to hear from others, he heard loud and clear "It's not your fault!" This surprised him. Though he knew intellectually that he was doing all he could to help in an impossible situation, emotionally he felt guilty and responsible. He fervently wanted to believe he could work miracles and judged himself for not being able to do so.

Arjun recognized that he needed to acknowledge his limits and lack of control. So he came up with the loving-kindness phrase "May I remember that I'm only human and doing the best I can."

He started repeating these two phrases over and over again:

> May I remember I'm only human and doing the best I can.
>
> May I live in peace and joy as often as possible.

At first Arjun didn't feel any different. He felt as down and burned out as ever. But the words felt like they fit him well. So he started to use them at work. He would pause outside a patient's room to repeat his loving-kindness phrases before entering. Eventually, he started to feel his own care and friendliness, and that brought him moments of peace and joy. He started being more supportive toward himself and did start remembering more often that he was a human being in an impossible job doing the best he could. Now, when Arjun is with a patient on a ventilator, he sometimes clasps their hands and silently offers them the wish "May your heart be peaceful." As if they can read his mind (though they are probably just reacting to his loving demeanor), patients often squeeze Arjun's hands in gratitude.

Although loving-kindness practice doesn't directly cultivate positive emotions, positive emotions are a natural by-product of goodwill. Loving-kindness does this without papering over difficult emotions. We're just opening our hearts, on purpose, to whatever comes. Other ways of opening our hearts and generating positive emotions without denying our pain are the practices of savoring and gratitude, which are the focus of the next chapter.

20

SMALL PLEASURES

Savoring the Good

The state of burnout is rife with negative thoughts and emotions: stress, hopelessness, numbness, overwhelm, and feelings of incompetence. Our exhausted bodies are not a happy place either. No wonder we eventually shut down in response to it all. Unfortunately, when we do, we toss out the proverbial baby with the bathwater. We don't just tune out negative emotions; we tune out the positive ones too.

The most devastating effect of burnout is arguably not the pain of exhaustion and depletion but the loss of enjoyment in life. We don't smile or laugh as often as we used to. We don't take pleasure in our work or in helping others the way we once did. We don't feel much of anything, including the joy of creativity or new discoveries. Our lives can become monotone and colorless.

Morgan (who uses the pronouns they/them) is a graphic artist in Seattle who used to love their job: the creativity and craftsmanship it required, the challenge of designing an image that inspired the viewer. It was fun, like drawing with crayons as a kid. But now Morgan works long hours at an advertising firm in a windowless office referred to as "the basement" (even though it's on the third floor). Clients' demand for images is nonstop and incredibly stressful. Upon arriving at work, Morgan is greeted by urgent emails demanding a progress update on projects with deadlines that are only days away. They worry about their ability to produce fresh digital images that can grab the attention of an increasingly jaded public (especially after some recent feedback saying that their submissions had been "a little stale").

But the thing that's really getting Morgan down is how boring the job has become. They go through the motions of the day like a robot, and back at home they sit in front of the TV in a similarly robotic state. Even though they have options—friends were always inviting Morgan to the local club to hear the latest new singer/songwriter, for instance—they can only see as far as the TV remote at the end of the day. Anything else is too much effort. So Morgan zones out until they fall asleep, gets up the next morning, and heads out for another day of work in the dreaded basement.

Healing burnout is not simply a matter of reversing the toll stress has taken. We need happiness and fun, not only to hasten the healing process but also to create a fulfilling life going forward. But this can seem like an impossibly tall order when things look so gray and gloomy.

THE NEGATIVITY BIAS

Unfortunately, our brains are hardwired to pay attention to problems due to an evolutionary hand-me-down called the *negativity bias*. Early on in human history, our ancestors who were on high alert to danger were more likely to survive and pass on their genes than those who relaxed in the cool breeze while a pack of hyenas snuck up on them. For this reason, modern-day brains are like Velcro for negative information and Teflon for positive information, as our friend Rick Hanson likes to say. If information doesn't have immediate survival value, we tend to ignore it.

The negativity bias is typically in overdrive when we're burned out. We narrowly focus on our stress, exhaustion, and sense of disconnection or incompetence to the point where we can see nothing else. We may not notice the fact that we're in relatively good health, or that we have a roof over our heads, or that we have people in our lives who care about us. Pleasure, joy, and happiness may feel alien as our perception of reality becomes more and more cynical.

Although we don't want to fake happiness, to be realistic we must pay attention to what's right as well as what's wrong in our life. The truth is that life is always a balance of light and dark, but because of the negativity bias of burnout, the light often gets relegated to the shadows.

ENTER POSITIVE PSYCHOLOGY

Since the turn of the millennium, the positive psychology movement has emphasized the need to intentionally cultivate positive thoughts and emotions to counteract the negativity bias. This bias used to prevail in the field of psychology as well, with most research being done on negative mind states like anxiety or depression. Now more and more research is being done on the benefits of positive states of mind like happiness and life satisfaction and the important role they play in mental health.

One of the pioneers of positive psychology, Barbara Frederickson, coined the term *broaden and build* to capture the benefits of positive emotions. Focusing on negative information narrows our attention on potential threats to our survival, whereas focusing on positive emotions broadens our perspective. When we acknowledge what's good about our lives, we feel safer and more relaxed. This allows us to be curious and recognize potential opportunities that may be just around the corner. Is that fresh water? Are those berries edible? When we expand our focus in this way, we encourage learning, growth, and play. We build our coping resources through innovation and creativity.

Even in the swamp of burnout, we can pay attention to positive experiences. We can take a moment to notice when a colleague flashes a warm smile, or when a job goes well, or when a meal is delicious. Small shifts in perspective can transform our internal landscape and restore balance, helping to energize and replenish us. This is not a case of putting on rose-colored glasses; it's a matter of looking at the world through clear lenses again. This clarity can help us take advantage of possible exit doors from burnout that were previously obscured. Maybe we could change our job, or speak with someone, or find creative ways to relax in our busy day. At the very least, we can counter the persistent drip drip drip of negativity that seems to have overtaken our lives.

Paying attention to positive experiences is not putting on rose-colored glasses but seeing through clear lenses again.

SELF-COMPASSION CREATES POSITIVE EMOTIONS

Research shows that one of the benefits of self-compassion is that it counteracts the negativity bias and generates positive emotions like happiness and life satisfaction. Compassion itself is a positive emotion—it gives us energy and helps us feel connected to others. Even though self-compassion (by definition) is a way of relating to suffering, self-compassion feels good. When we are kind to ourselves and remind ourselves that we aren't alone, we experience positive feelings of care and belonging in addition to our feelings of distress. It's an alchemical process, transforming pain into an experience in which our hearts are open and flowing with love.

Self-compassion is considered part of the positive psychology movement because it's a strength and resource that enhances our lives. Studies indicate that self-compassionate people tend to be more hopeful and optimistic than those who are harsh toward themselves. They are more open and curious and oriented toward growth and learning. Researchers have also found that people who practice loving-kindness, as described in the last chapter, feel more love, joy, gratitude, contentment, hope, pride, interest, amusement, and awe. By using the tools provided in this book to counter burnout, you are automatically countering the negativity bias. But there are two other ways to intentionally cultivate positive emotions that we teach as part of the MSC program: gratitude and savoring.

GRATITUDE

Gratitude is a matter of noticing and appreciating the gifts we're given. It involves acknowledging the many factors, large and small, that contribute to what's good in our life. We may be grateful for the people who make things better—like family and friends or public servants like first responders or educators or poll workers. We may be grateful for our health, our ability to see, speak, smell, hear, and move. Gratitude may be inspired by features of our culture like art and music, literature, science, medicine, or technological advances like electricity, cars, phones, or computers.

When we're grateful, we recognize the interdependence of things, dispelling the illusion that we're separate. We acknowledge the myriad causes and conditions that have come together to create our lives as we know them. People often think of gratitude as being nice, like writing a thank-you note. This diminishes how profound it is.

> **Gratitude is the wisdom of the heart.**

Practicing gratitude is really the cultivation of wisdom. It's about seeing the complexity of the world through the eyes of love.

Gratitude is also a positive emotion. Notice how instantly your mood is transformed when you switch from complaining about how your feet hurt to being grateful for the fact that you can walk (implicitly acknowledging that many people can't). This isn't an effort to brush off or deny the fact that your feet hurt, but it places things in a larger context. It broadens your perspective so that you simultaneously acknowledge that (1) your feet hurt and (2) you're grateful you can walk. In this way gratitude allows us to move beyond the narrow focus on what's broken and expand our focus to include appreciation for what works.

Not surprisingly, research shows that a regular practice of gratitude lifts people up, increasing emotional and physical well-being. It increases happiness, hope, vitality, and life satisfaction. In particular, studies suggest that individuals in high-stress jobs who have higher levels of gratitude experience lower levels of burnout—particularly in terms of exhaustion, disengagement, and cynicism.

So how to practice gratitude? One simple method is to spend a few minutes every night before going to sleep and think of ten things—one for each finger—that you're grateful for. It could be obvious things like your family or taken-for-granted things like hot water, zippers, or written language. Intentionally focusing on those aspects of your life that are good, that aren't part of the experience of burnout, can prevent you from being so overwhelmed by negative thoughts and emotions. It doesn't take much time but can produce a dramatic shift in your emotional outlook and energy levels.

SAVORING

Savoring may be called *permission to enjoy*. Savoring is experiential and involves consciously taking pleasure in things. It means recognizing the experiences that give us joy, allowing ourselves to be drawn in by them, lingering with them so that we connect with the good feelings they generate, and then letting them go. Think of eating your favorite ice cream: let's say it's chocolate gelato. If you do it on autopilot while scrolling on your phone, you might not even taste it. But if you savor the experience, you pay full attention to the smell, texture, and flavor, allowing yourself to relish each bite. You eat slowly so you prolong the delight and then move on feeling satisfied once you've finished.

When we're burned out, there's so much pressure on us to rush through everything that doesn't contribute to getting our work done that we stop taking pleasure in life. Savoring counteracts this pressure. It's easy and requires just a shift in intention. Can you find moments in your day to mindfully take pleasure in simple things like these?

- ❑ Softly caress your hands and notice the tingles on your skin (you can try this right now).
- ❑ Look outside your window, see if there's anything beautiful, and allow yourself to really enjoy its beauty.
- ❑ Eat something you like, savoring the taste, smell, and texture of your food.
- ❑ Play with your child or your pet, giving yourself permission to have fun.
- ❑ Take a warm bath or shower, luxuriating in the hot water running over your naked body.
- ❑ Look at some photos of a vacation you took and linger with the memories of something especially wonderful from the trip.

There is something pleasurable about most experiences if we take the time to seek it out and linger with the joy it provides. It's not a waste of time—quite the opposite. Especially when we're burned out, these small moments of pleasure can be a lifesaver and provide an essential antidote to the darkness generated by our negativity bias. The following tool can help you start paying attention to and begin to savor what's pleasurable in your environment, even if it's been shrouded by the cloud of burnout.

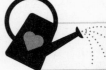

SELF-COMPASSION TOOL 20
Sense and Savor Walk

This practice can be done anywhere—at a park or while walking to work or in your backyard. While it's best done outdoors in nature, you can also do it in an indoor space that is attractive or interesting.

✦ Take fifteen minutes to amble about silently, noticing and savoring any beautiful or interesting objects you come into contact with—the bark on a tree, the clouds in the sky, a painting that's hung on a wall, a child holding a parent's hand.

+ Play with perspective, sometimes focusing on small things like an ant, at other times focusing on big things like the skyline.

+ Allow yourself to be drawn into and then to savor each object using all your senses—sight, smell, sound, touch . . . maybe even taste.

+ The goal is not to "try" to enjoy yourself or to make anything happen. Instead, each time you find something delightful or pleasant, let yourself be drawn into it. Really savor it. Feel the texture of a stick or listen to the crinkle of a leaf. *Give yourself over* to the experience as if it were the only thing that existed in the world.

+ When you lose interest and would like to discover something new, let go and wait until you discover something else that is attractive and delightful to you. Be like a bumblebee floating from one flower to another. When you feel satiated with one experience, go to another.

+ How many beautiful, attractive, or inspiring things do you notice while you're walking? Do you enjoy the scent of freshly cut grass, the warm sun, the shape of a stone, a smiling face, the song of a bird, the feeling of the earth under your feet?

+ Take your time, move slowly, and see what comes.

+ After the fifteen minutes are up, see how your mood may have changed. Did you notice anything new or inspiring? Do you feel uplifted?

+ You don't have to stop savoring after fifteen minutes, of course. If you like, you can do this practice for the rest of your life.

When Morgan first heard about the sense and savor walk from a friend, they were intrigued. Morgan lived a twenty-minute walk away from their office, so they tried doing this practice while walking home after work. They noticed that there was a crabapple tree in full bloom, and marveled at the deep pink of the blossoms and the luxurious spread of its branches. They picked up a stone and were surprised by the fact that it had little sparkly flakes in it that reflected light when held up to the sun. They were inspired by the architecture of an old building created in the Art Deco period. Morgan felt like a kid again, noticing things as if for the first time. Even after five minutes of savoring in this way, they felt lighter.

After a few weeks of practicing savoring, Morgan woke up one morning with tears in their eyes and proclaimed out loud, "I forgot what joy felt like." It wasn't that they had suddenly fallen in love, gotten a puppy, or won the lottery. What reminded Morgan was noticing the breeze gently blowing the curtains, bringing the gift of warm early-morning sunshine.

What really impressed Morgan was the boost in creativity that savoring practice gave them. Whenever they were stuck in designing an image, they would look around their environment for inspiration: a beautiful photograph on their desk, the smell of the Thai food their colleague was eating, the clever quirkiness of their Felix the Cat watch. This simple act of focusing and enjoying something pleasant would often kick-start the creative process and brought a playful quality back to it.

Although Morgan's work remained stressful and the pressure was still tiring, they felt like they had a better perspective on it all. They started to prioritize having fun as an essential part of their routine and took up the offer of going out to listen to some good music. Morgan had brought some color back into their life or, more accurately, they had started to notice the colors that were already there. It made a huge difference to their happiness and well-being, and Morgan credits savoring practice for pulling them out of burnout.

Although most people intuitively see the value of practicing savoring or gratitude, usually we focus on things that we appreciate in the environment or in other people. When we're burned out, however, we need to turn our focus inward as well, so that we learn to savor and be grateful for our own positive qualities. In the next chapter we explore the practice of self-appreciation, an essential counterpart to the practice of self-compassion in which we rediscover our own goodness.

21

KNOWING OUR STRENGTHS

The Practice of Self-Appreciation

The negativity bias—seeing what's wrong rather than what's right—operates especially powerfully when we look at ourselves. When we gaze into the mirror, we tend to see what we don't like, not what we *do* like. This is true for everyone, but add burnout to the mix and that mirror becomes especially distorted. One of the key features of burnout is feeling incompetent. The negative emotions we experience from work stress color our perceptions of ourselves. And the sense of brokenness that defines burnout exacerbates the natural tendency of our brains to zero in on our weaknesses, so we may perceive ourselves as hopelessly flawed and inadequate. Although there is value in considering where we could make changes and improvements (see Chapter 18), overdoing it leaves us with a skewed picture of reality. We need to acknowledge our gifts as well as our deficits to view our capabilities clearly and accurately.

Imagine getting a performance evaluation and receiving sixteen positive comments (hard work, perseverance, loyalty, intelligence, humor, maturity, etc.) and one negative one (has difficulty meeting deadlines). You're likely to pass over the positive remarks quickly—they're not problems that need to be fixed—and obsess about the one negative comment. Ruminating on your shortcomings may lead you to see yourself as a screw-up who can't do anything right, even though your performance review was overwhelmingly positive.

Having tunnel vision focused on weaknesses works directly against growth and learning. It inhibits your ability to access the accurate feedback and information needed to take effective action. It also makes it harder to build on your strengths and use them to your advantage.

Jamal has eight hard years under his belt working for the Chicago Fire Department as an EMT (emergency medical technician). He's skilled at what he does and has saved many lives. Despite the twelve-hour shifts and constant action, Jamal is usually calm, sharp, and brave in even the worst emergencies. He knows how to crack a joke at just the right time to ease tension. The other EMTs instinctively look to Jamal for reassurance and support when they start to lose it on a call; catching his eye and getting an encouraging nod helps them get back to saving lives.

Lately, though, Jamal's calm facade has developed some cracks. He's been having trouble sleeping and has been experiencing flashbacks from a gruesome car accident that killed an entire family. He has a hard time focusing and has been unusually nervous and anxious. The department counselor thinks Jamal is suffering from burnout caused by posttraumatic stress and has recommended that he stop going out into the field, at least for the time being.

That idea horrifies Jamal even more than his nightmares. He would feel like a coward if he couldn't be on the front lines. He wants to be out there saving lives, but his shot nerves tell a different story. Jamal feels like he's got nothing to offer the department anymore and is thinking of quitting, completely overlooking his intelligence and leadership skills.

CELEBRATING OUR POSITIVE QUALITIES

When we're compassionate toward our perceived inadequacies, we prevent ourselves from spiraling into negative mind states like depression. But self-compassion isn't enough to pull us out of burnout. We also need to actively acknowledge our strengths and competencies. An important corollary of self-compassion is self-appreciation, which involves focusing on and celebrating our positive qualities. Think of self-appreciation as gratitude and savoring turned inward.

Self-appreciation involves turning gratitude and savoring inward.

Self-appreciation means we honor the part of our glass that is half full as well as having compassion for the part that is half empty. We recognize what's *not* broken.

Acknowledging the good qualities that we've overlooked can help us recover from burnout by reminding us of the various internal resources that are available to us. If we don't acknowledge our strong points and think only about our weak points, how do we know what we're capable of? How can we recover if we can't identify the best foot to put forward?

According to the broaden-and-build theory of positive emotions discussed in the last chapter, focusing on our strengths allows us to move beyond a narrow focus on problems so that we can take advantage of opportunities we may have overlooked. Consider Jamal, who is thinking about quitting the fire department because he can't go out into the field anymore. If he were to appreciate his strengths, he might pursue a management position at the department that would be a good fit for him. But focusing on his own positive qualities makes Jamal squirm.

Even though it seems like it should be enjoyable to revel in our good qualities, it's often uncomfortable. Do you cringe or blush when someone compliments you, stammering out a protest? Does acknowledging your strengths make you feel like a fraud? Does it make you feel weird to think about your good qualities? If so, you aren't alone.

WHY IS SELF-APPRECIATION SO DIFFICULT?

Ironically, it can be harder for us to appreciate the positive aspects of ourselves than to have compassion for the negatives. This is not just the negativity bias at work. Another reason it's challenging is because self-appreciation is so unfamiliar. We're used to feeling bad about ourselves, and the cloak of inadequacy may have become as comfortable as a well-worn sweater. Incompetence can be so central to our sense of self that focusing on what we do well and why we're valuable can feel frightening. We don't want to let go of the devil we know, so our negative self-image fights to survive. But if we aren't familiar with our strengths, how are we going to use them effectively when needed?

When our strengths feel alien to us, it's harder to call them up when we need their help.

Another factor inhibiting self-appreciation is that we're afraid it puts us on a pedestal we might fall from. If we're on the floor already, we can't fall any farther. If I acknowledge my wisdom, diligence, or integrity, I risk disappointing

Identifying Your Strengths

A number of character strengths studied in the field of positive psychology appear to be valued across cultures. Do any of the following describe you?

- ❑ Creativity: Thinking up novel and productive ways to conceptualize or do things
- ❑ Curiosity: Taking an interest in experience for its own sake; exploring and discovering
- ❑ Open-mindedness: Examining things from all sides; not jumping to conclusions
- ❑ Love of learning: Mastering new skills, topics, and bodies of knowledge
- ❑ Wisdom: Looking at the world in ways that make sense to yourself and to other people
- ❑ Courage: Not shrinking from challenges; speaking up for what is right
- ❑ Perseverance: Persisting in a course of action despite obstacles
- ❑ Integrity: Speaking the truth; acting sincerely; taking responsibility for your actions
- ❑ Love and care: Valuing close relations and intimacy; being kind and helpful
- ❑ Social intelligence: Knowing how to fit into different social situations
- ❑ Teamwork: Making contributions and being loyal to a group or team
- ❑ Fairness: Treating all people the same according to principles of justice
- ❑ Leadership: Organizing group activities and inspiring others

myself and others when I don't display these traits. We confuse acknowledging our good qualities with saying that we are perfect and never make mistakes. This is a misperception. The reality is we get some things right some of the time and some things wrong some of the time; that's the human condition. Both the light and the dark are true.

One of the biggest reasons people feel uncomfortable with self-appreciation is that they confuse it with being conceited. Jamal certainly fell prey to this notion. "My parents taught me not to brag," he would often say. Born to a family that valued humility and modesty, Jamal is humble to a fault. When his coworkers praise his calm demeanor in the midst of chaos or tell him he's a role model, he typically waves them off or makes a joke because he doesn't want to come off as full of himself. But being conceited means believing we're better than others. Self-appreciation simply acknowledges that we have strengths as well as weaknesses, just like everyone else. Humility that refuses to recognize our good qualities is as false as arrogance that refuses to recognize our shortcomings.

To complicate matters, we all harbor an innate desire to be loved and to be special. As philosopher and psychologist William James said, "The deepest principle in human nature is the craving to be appreciated." But it's lonely at the top! When we confuse self-appreciation with egotism, it creates a sense of separation that we both want (to be special) and don't want (to feel isolated from others). This internal conflict is exhausting and can contribute to stress and burnout.

It's important to recognize that self-appreciation is an inside job. It has to do with how we relate to ourselves in our own minds and hearts, not necessarily what we say to others. We don't need to boast about our good qualities to others, especially if it might come across the wrong way. But we shouldn't swing in the opposite direction and pretend our strengths don't exist either. Ideally, we can be our authentic selves around others, which includes acknowledging the ways we excel.

As Marianne Williamson writes in her book *A Return to Love*:

> Your playing small does not serve the world.

> There is nothing enlightened about shrinking so that other people won't feel insecure around you.

We are all meant to shine, as children do . . .

And as we let our own light shine,

we unconsciously give other people permission to do the same.

We're more effective at overcoming burnout when we choose coping strategies that are in line with our personal strengths. For instance, pausing and taking time to consider all possible options before making work-related changes may be more beneficial for those who are good at strategic thinking than for those who are better at taking bold action. For this reason, it's worth considering what our own personal strengths are.

APPRECIATING OUR STRENGTHS WITH THE THREE COMPONENTS OF SELF-COMPASSION

The three core elements of self-compassion—mindfulness, common humanity, and self-kindness—each play a role when appreciating our strengths. In combination, they allow us to acknowledge our capacities and build on them in a way that refills our cup and helps us recover from burnout.

Mindful awareness means seeing our positive qualities as they are, without ignoring or exaggerating what is. Practicing mindfulness can free us from the automatic responses of the brain such as the negativity bias so that we don't take our strengths for granted. As with self-compassion, mindfulness is the first step of self-appreciation: we need to *notice* what's good before we can appreciate it. When we're exhausted and depressed, it can seem daunting to notice our good qualities, but it requires only a few moments to intentionally acknowledge the truth of what's working in addition to what's broken.

Recognizing common humanity takes the "self" out of self-appreciation, making it feel more comfortable and connected. It prevents feelings of superiority and identifies our strengths as part of the human condition. Everybody has good qualities, some of which may be uncommon (such as an outstanding intellect or physical prowess) and some that may be more common (such as caring about our family). Also, recognizing our common humanity allows us to become aware of other people or events that helped us develop our good qualities. When framed in terms of our shared humanity, self-appreciation helps us feel like part of a larger whole.

Kindness is what moves us to honor our own goodness, just as we would with a friend we care about. There's nothing like feeling truly seen, and self-appreciation allows us to be seen and loved in all our glory. Without denying our imperfection, we celebrate the unique qualities that make us who we are. When we're drained and burned out, this form of kindness can feel like a cool drink of water in a parched desert. Recognizing and appreciating our strengths energizes and inspires us, exactly what we need to take on the challenge of burnout.

The following exercise will help you discover and appreciate your strengths. Even though you may not be performing at your best because you're burned out, you still have positive qualities that are worthy of acknowledging and appreciating. Some people find this practice difficult, especially those who suffered from childhood trauma or were raised in an environment where it was "bad" to feel proud of themselves. If this practice produces backdraft (see Chapter 7), please be compassionate with yourself. It may be a signal that this is a fruitful practice for you, to be done slowly, with patience.

SELF-COMPASSION TOOL 21
Appreciating Your Strengths

+ Take two or three deep breaths as you settle and center yourself. Put your hands on your heart or use some other supportive touch as a gesture of warmth and care.

+ Think of some of the key strengths that you display in your work life. Please take your time and be honest. Remember that you aren't saying you *always* display these qualities or that you're better than others. You're simply acknowledging that this, too, is true.

+ Consider each of these strengths, one by one, and offer yourself an inner nod of appreciation for having these gifts. Let yourself feel your own goodness.

+ Notice if there is any discomfort as you think about your strengths and make space for them, allowing your experience to be just as it is.

- ✦ Now try expanding the circle of appreciation. Are there any people or experiences that helped you develop your strengths? Maybe friends, parents, teachers, books, or educational institutions that had a positive impact on you? Maybe your culture or history? As each of these helpful influences come to mind, please send them some gratitude and appreciation as well.

- ✦ You may have had negative role models that also reminded you of what you *didn't* want to become. That, too, was a kind of contribution.

- ✦ Let yourself savor, just for this moment, feeling good about yourself—let it really soak in.

- ✦ If you had difficulty with this exercise, that's okay too. It takes some time. You can still offer yourself appreciation for your efforts.

Jamal did a version of this exercise, which was recommended to him by the department counselor. It took a while to settle into the exercise at the beginning, but it felt good when he gently rubbed his chest as a supportive gesture.

The next step was challenging—identifying key strengths. Whenever Jamal tried to list something, he'd come up with a sarcastic or silly response, like "I'm a really good dancer" (his wife could attest to the fact that he is not). When he tried to call up a true strength, like perseverance, he started arguing with himself. "But I can't stick with it anymore. I'm thinking of quitting!" Then he remembered that the quality didn't have to always be there; typically he did display perseverance. He also realized he had other good qualities—courage, teamwork, social intelligence, and leadership.

As soon as Jamal started to feel some appreciation for his strengths, feelings of shame arose. He remembered how his mom would scold him whenever he exhibited anything even close to "bragging." He realized how difficult it was to have his light dimmed in this way. Jamal had to take this exercise very slowly, stopping when he felt overwhelmed, giving himself compassion, and going back to it when he felt more settled (perseverance really was one of his strengths).

What made a big difference was the instruction to appreciate all the people who helped him develop his strengths. There were so many: his history professor in college, a brilliant teacher; his grandfather, who was active in the civil rights movement; his good friend Tanisha, who was always so supportive; his favorite film, *Black Panther*. Once he expanded the circle of appreciation in this way, it became a lot easier for him to savor and be grateful for his own goodness.

This practice helped him realize that he could still have a place at the Chicago Fire Department. He had strong leadership skills, and he loved to bring out the best in team members. He decided he would talk to Human Resources about applying for a supervising or managing officer position.

When you give yourself permission to acknowledge your *whole* self—the good as well as the bad—you open the door to living a fuller, more authentic life. Self-appreciation is not selfish, self-centered, or egotistical. It's a form of wisdom that acknowledges what's true. We all yearn to know and believe in our own goodness, especially when we're lost in the dark cloud of burnout. The practice of self-appreciation allows our sun to shine.

With all the tools you've acquired in this book, hopefully you've started to see that emerging from burnout is fully possible for you. Each person's path will be unique, and we should expect ourselves to stumble—often. This isn't a problem, as long as we have the practice of self-compassion to support us. In the final chapter, we explore how to embrace the process of stumbling and getting back up again as we move on from burnout and go forward into the rest of our lives.

22

MOVING FORWARD

Becoming a Compassionate Mess

You did it! You've arrived at the last chapter of this book. Not bad for someone who's burned out. Chances are you've been through many ups and downs along the way. Some chapters probably made sense to you and others not so much. There might have been some days when you thought you were over burnout, only to be thrown back into the pits. And how do you feel now about your ability to be self-compassionate? Optimistic? Discouraged? Reassured?

Remember Jacquie, the critical care nurse, from Chapter 1? When we left her, she was slumped in the front seat of her car, hardly able to move after yet another grueling shift at the hospital.

Fortunately for Jacquie, her hospital started offering the Self-Compassion for Healthcare Communities (SCHC) course. She decided to sign up for it since a dear friend said she'd do it with her. Learning about self-compassion turned on a light bulb in her mind. It made a lot of sense to her that she was going to burn out if she didn't give herself the same compassion she gives to her patients. Jacquie decided to give self-compassion practice a try with whatever energy she still had left in her.

During the course Jacquie saw some positive changes in her life. For starters, it was a relief to learn that being burned out is not a sign of failure—it's a sign of being human. Jacquie also learned to calm herself by feeling the soles of her feet, especially when she felt emotionally overwhelmed, and by letting herself be rocked by the rhythm of her breathing. What really helped Jacquie, though, was learning to talk in a kinder, more supportive way with herself, just as she typically spoke with her patients. That little U-turn made all the difference to Jacquie. Her sleep also improved during the course, and she found herself going to work more refreshed.

Shortly after the course ended, however, she had a setback. Jacquie began waking up at 3:00 A.M. again, fretting about the day ahead. Jacquie also noticed that her self-talk had resumed its hard edge: "What's the matter with you? You can't even get self-compassion right!" Jacquie shared her despair with the friend who had taken the course with her, who suggested that she treat herself with warmth and kindness simply *because* she was feeling so frustrated and disappointed. "Ohhhh, right!" Jacquie exclaimed. "*That's* self-compassion!" From then on, Jacquie's practice was steadier.

STAGES OF PROGRESS

The path to self-compassion takes twists and turns but typically goes through three stages. We start out hoping and expecting that some good will come of our journey—that we'll feel better, our life will improve, or we'll somehow become a better person. That's the first stage, the *striving* stage. It works for a while, as Jacquie discovered during her self-compassion course.

Sooner or later, however, everyone becomes disillusioned. The *disillusionment* stage sets in when we come to the awkward realization that we're still suffering; maybe less so, but we're still the same person with the same problems. This phase is like the end of infatuation in a romantic relationship, when the love bubble is pricked and we realize that the person who was supposed to be the answer to all our dreams is—horror of horrors—a flawed human being! It can be even worse when we practice self-compassion because *we're* the disappointment. Anyhow, that was how Jacquie felt when her sleeplessness returned and she thought she was a failure at self-compassion.

The disillusionment stage of self-compassion is actually a sign of progress. It doesn't feel that way when we're in the thick of it, but we wouldn't feel disillusioned if we didn't already have some successful self-compassion mileage behind us. Disillusionment is a gift, because it makes room for genuine self-compassion to arise. How? Do you remember reading about how resistance to burnout makes burnout worse in the long run? When we're at the disillusionment stage, the problem is not *what* we're practicing but *why* we're practicing.

After a while we unconsciously start to practice self-compassion as a way to get rid of bad feelings, which is nothing more than a slick new form of resistance. The solution to this problem (given in Chapter 9) is the "central paradox of self-compassion": *when we suffer, we practice self-compassion not to feel better but because we feel bad*. This crazy paradox is an invitation to love ourselves up, just as we are. No strategy—just kindness, like caring for a child with the flu just because the child feels lousy.

Jack Kornfield put it beautifully: "The point . . . isn't to perfect yourself, but to perfect your *love*." That's *radical acceptance*—stage three. Most of our self-improvement strategies eventually fail because they're based on resistance rather than acceptance. There's a subtle form of aggression in them because, at the outset, the assumption is that we aren't good enough as we are. Radical acceptance puts self-improvement on an entirely new footing. Rather than improving our "selves"—after all, our worth is unconditional—we focus on improving our behaviors and situations as an act of compassionate motivation (see Chapter 18). Fierce self-compassion inspires us to make the changes needed to be happy and fulfilled in life not out of a sense of inadequacy but out of love. But this happens only when we're disillusioned by business as usual.

> **Self-compassion practice has three stages—striving, disillusionment, and radical acceptance.**

After Jacquie's friend reminded her of the central paradox, she started relating to her insomnia in an entirely new way. Instead of struggling to get to sleep, she put her hand on her heart and hummed softly until she drifted off. Jacquie also learned to say a gentle but firm "No, not now" to the inner voice that was criticizing her for not doing better, and she replaced the self-criticism with words of support: "You can do this. I believe in you!"

THE PATH OF LEAST RESISTANCE

The big surprise for Jacquie was how much easier her life became when she remembered radical acceptance—accepting herself and her pain. Jacquie discovered that her passion for her work as a critical care nurse gradually returned when she learned to support herself just as she did others. Like falling in love or falling asleep, Jacquie let herself fall into self-compassion.

At first Jacquie had worried that by letting in the pain of burnout she would become emotionally overwhelmed. This didn't happen because she had learned to be kind to herself when she felt pain, not just to open to the pain, which gave her more strength. When Jacquie was on the edge of overwhelm, she asked herself the quintessential self-compassion question, "Honey, what do you need?" Usually the answer was something simple, such as taking a few breaths, taking a break, or even occasionally taking an entire day off from work.

Another concern that arose for Jacquie was that if she accepted herself as she was, she would be less likely to make needed changes in her life. Well, that didn't happen either. Jacquie noticed that she started making smarter choices when she put compassion first. As the famous psychologist Carl Rogers once wrote, "the curious paradox is that when I accept myself as I am . . . change seems to come about almost unnoticed."

Did Jacquie arrive at the stage of radical acceptance and stay there forever? Of course not. The conditions of our lives are continually changing, resistance springs eternal, and inner change happens gradually. We cycle through the three stages of self-compassion—striving, disillusionment, and radical acceptance— over and over again. For example, if we recognize that we're truly accepting, we will instinctively try to hang on to the good feelings of that state, which triggers another round of striving. Conversely, when we notice that we're striving or disillusioned and we respond with compassion, we're back into radical acceptance. The good news is that, over time, we spend more and more time in radical acceptance.

BECOMING A COMPASSIONATE MESS

The practice of self-compassion doesn't mean that we stop trying to achieve our goals, but it does mean that we stop basing our worth on success and drop unrealistic expectations of perfection. We make a cheeky statement in the MSC program that often stops people in their tracks: "The goal of practice is simply to be a compassionate mess."

If you're a perfectionist, this statement is probably making your heart palpitate right now. "What? Our goal is to be a mess?" Allow us to clarify. The goal of practice is not to become a mess. (That won't happen anyway— remember that self-compassion practice doesn't lower our standards; it just makes them easier to achieve.) The statement means that when we feel like a mess—making mistakes, failing, struggling, confused, overwhelmed (that is, fully human!)—our goal is to bring *compassion* to the mess.

> **The goal of practice is simply to be a compassionate mess.**

Over time, the "compassionate mess" agenda becomes a way of life. We're more able to accept our mistakes and learn from them. Instead of trying to get it right all the time, we develop a keen interest in meeting our failures and shortcomings with a tender, supportive, open heart. After a while, living from this place of open-heartedness becomes the most important thing for us. We learn to linger in the feelings of loving, connected presence that any moment of self-compassion brings, and we realize that this is the happiness we've been seeking all along.

WHAT SHOULD I DO NOW?

At this point, you might be thinking, "Okay, I get it. Self-compassion can help me shift my mindset for the better. But a big part of my burnout is the situation I'm in. What should I do?" This is when we need to bring in wisdom. Wisdom refers to understanding the complexity of a situation and finding our way through. If you work in a health care setting as Jacquie does, the problem may be systemic—not enough nurses treating too many patients. What should Jacquie do? The answer depends on many factors—Jacquie's talents, how much time and energy she has, her role at the hospital, her values, her connections, her financial resources, and so forth. The only thing that's certain is that no one would be in a better position than Jacquie to know *what* to do and *when* to do it.

When Jacquie's mind started getting a little clearer, she decided she wanted to fight for better working conditions. There's strength in numbers, she reasoned, so she joined her health care union and eventually became one of their most vocal advocates when the union went on strike. Taking action in this way felt just right for Jacquie—the perfect combination of wisdom and compassion. So, if you're wondering what *your* next move should be, now that you've learned self-compassion, please take your time and consider all the factors at play in your own situation and then take action when the time feels right. What does *your* wisdom suggest you do?

PRACTICING FOR LIFE

Each of the preceding twenty-one chapters has closed with a self-compassion practice, or tool. There's one remaining practice—the rest of your life! It's up to you to figure out how to best bring self-compassion to your unique and precious life. In the box is a list of the tools that you've acquired in this book. Can you identify two or three self-compassion tools that seem to have had the greatest

Your Self-Compassion Tools

1. Self-compassion assessment
2. How would you treat a friend or colleague who was feeling burned out?
3. A self-compassionate letter for burnout
4. Craft a self-compassion reminder
5. Supportive touch
6. Tender self-compassion break
7. Soles of the feet
8. Affectionate breathing
9. Reducing resistance to work-related stress
10. Being with difficult emotions related to burnout
11. Compassion with equanimity
12. Letting go of the need to be perfect
13. Finding your compassionate voice
14. Protective self-compassion break
15. Getting comfortable with boundaries
16. Providing self-compassion break
17. Discovering your core values
18. Motivating self-compassion break
19. Finding loving-kindness phrases
20. Sense and savor walk
21. Appreciating your strengths

impact? Trust your intuition. The best teacher of self-compassion is always yourself.

Maybe you modified a tool in a way that made more sense to you? Perhaps you created an entirely new practice while you were reading this book? Please note any ways that you might like to practice, going forward, whenever you need a bit of self-compassion.

Practice is essential, but remember, if it's a struggle, it's not self-compassion. The self-compassion practice you're most likely to do is one that's relatively pleasant and easy. You don't want it to feel like work, because more work is the last thing you need when you feel burned out. Sometimes a practice is pleasant at first but becomes bland or mechanical over time. Then ask yourself, "Is there anything I can let go of that would make this easier?" For example, if you enjoy affectionate breathing and later on it feels like a chore, has it become unnecessarily complicated? What would happen if you just let yourself be rocked gently by the rhythm of your breathing (Chapter 8)? Similarly, if your loving-kindness phrases (Chapter 19) have lost their magic, try asking yourself, "What would I really love to hear someone say to me right now?" and say *that* to yourself. There's always a way to restore your practice to its original shine.

Be merciful with yourself. That may mean lowering your expectations of self-compassion practice. Self-compassion is good *will* training, not good feelings training. Although it's easier to practice when it's pleasant, you don't have to feel good as an outcome of practice to indicate it's working. The *wish* to be self-compassionate is enough. When you ask yourself, "What do I need?" you're already practicing self-compassion. In answer to that question, it's amazing how many different activities increase self-compassion. Research shows that self-compassion can increase through owning a dog, doing yoga, immersing yourself in nature, going to therapy, learning mindfulness, giving support to others, or taking a long walk. Just about anything we do for ourselves with a compassionate heart will probably increase our self-compassion.

How will you know if your practice is working? When perfectionism loses its grip and you let yourself be a slow learner, and when you move at your own pace and take it one day at a time, that's a good sign. When you're not on top of your game, and you *still* feel okay about yourself, you're probably making progress. And when you know that you're *enough*—your body is enough, your emotions are enough, your intellect is enough—just as you are, in this moment, you're definitely on your way. When you *love* yourself, no matter what, you've arrived.

We thank you from the bottom of our hearts for taking this journey with us. May the suffering of burnout be a doorway to compassion for you, and may your self-compassionate presence be a gift to everyone you meet.

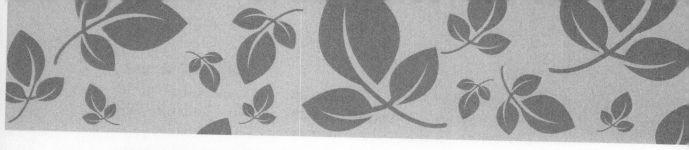

RESOURCES

CENTER FOR MINDFUL SELF-COMPASSION

https://centerformsc.org

- Guided recordings of self-compassion practices
- Self-compassion information and blog
- Online training programs for beginners, advanced practitioners, and professionals
- Information on Self-Compassion for Healthcare Communities program

Social Media

- Instagram: centerformindfulselfcompassion
- Facebook: CenterforMSC
- LinkedIn: center-for-mindful-self-compassion
- YouTube: CenterforMindfulSelfCompassion

KRISTIN NEFF

www.self-compassion.org

- The Self-Compassion Community (membership subscription)
- Information on self-compassion
- Guided meditations and exercises
- Test your own self-compassion level
- Library of self-compassion research
- Upcoming talks and workshops

Social Media

- Instagram: neffselfcompassion
- Facebook: selfcompassion
- X: self_compassion
- YouTube: NeffKristin

CHRISTOPHER GERMER

www.chrisgermer.com

- Audio and video presentations
- Guided meditations and exercises
- Self-compassion in psychotherapy
- Upcoming talks and workshops

Social Media

- Instagram: christophergermerphd
- Facebook: christophergermerphd
- X: chrisgermerphd
- YouTube: ChristopherGermer

BOOKS

Germer, C. (2009). *The mindful path to self-compassion: Freeing yourself from destructive thoughts and emotions.* New York: Guilford Press.

Germer, C., & Neff, K. (2019). *Teaching the Mindful Self-Compassion program: A guide for professionals.* New York: Guilford Press.

Germer, C., & Siegel, R. (2012). *Wisdom and compassion in psychotherapy: Deepening mindfulness in clinical practice.* New York: Guilford Press.

Neff, K. (2011). *Self-compassion: The proven power of being kind to yourself.* New York: William Morrow.

Neff, K. (2021). *Fierce self-compassion: How women can harness kindness to speak up, claim their power, and thrive.* New York: Harper.

Neff, K., & Germer, C. (2018). *The Mindful Self-Compassion workbook: A proven way to accept yourself, build inner strength, and thrive.* New York: Guilford Press.

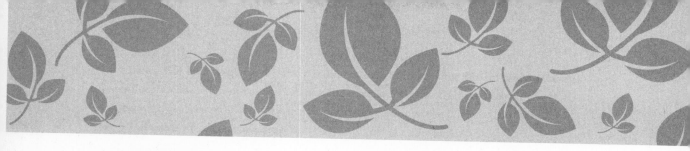

NOTES

INTRODUCTION

PAGE 3   **"published the first study examining the link between self-compassion and well-being":** Neff, K. D. (2003). The development and validation of a scale to measure self-compassion. *Self and Identity, 2*(3), 223–250.

CHAPTER 1. WHEN YOUR CUP RUNS DRY: THE CAUSES AND CONSEQUENCES OF BURNOUT

PAGE 6   **"scientifically proven to increase self-compassion and reduce burnout":** Delaney, M. C. (2018). Caring for the caregivers: Evaluation of the effect of an eight-week pilot Mindful Self-Compassion (MSC) training program on nurses' compassion fatigue and resilience. *PLOS ONE, 13*(11), e0207261.

PAGE 6   **"Burnout is typically defined by these three symptoms":** Maslach, C., & Jackson, S. E. (1981). The measurement of experienced burnout. *Journal of Organizational Behavior, 2*(2), 99–113.

PAGE 6   **"'Burnout' was coined in 1974 by clinical psychologist Herbert Freudenberger":** Freudenberger, H. J. (1974). Staff burn-out. *Journal of Social Issues, 30*(1), 159–165.

PAGE 6   **"between one-third and three-quarters of people worldwide are burned out":** Taylor, H. (2023, June). 50+ burnout statistics that will shock you into action. Retrieved from *www.runn.io/blog/burnout-statistics#how-common-is-employee-burnout.*

   Spring Health. (2020, December). Burnout nation. Retrieved from *https://lp.springhealth.com/burnout-nation.*

   Future Forum. (2023, February). Future Forum winter snapshot. Retrieved from *https://futureforum.com/research/future-forum-pulse-winter-2022-2023-snapshot.*

Gallup (2023). The state of the global workplace: 2023 report. Retrieved from *www.gallup.com/workplace/506879/state-global-workplace-2023-report.aspx*.

PAGE 8   **"Burnout can cause physical problems"**: Shirom, A., Melamed, S., Toker, S., Berliner, S., & Shapira, I. (2005). Burnout and health review: Current knowledge and future research directions. *International Review of Industrial and Organizational Psychology, 20*(1), 269–308.

PAGE 9   **"many are exiting due to burnout, especially health care workers"**: Doctors not the only ones feeling burned out. (2023, March 31). *Harvard Gazette*. Retrieved from *https://news.harvard.edu/gazette/story/2023/03/covid-burnout-hitting-all-levels-of-health-care-workforce*.

PAGE 9   **"scientists have linked burnout with several identifiable factors"**: Maslach, C., Schaufeli, W. B., & Leiter, M. P. (2001). Job burnout. *Annual Review of Psychology, 52*(1), 397–422.

PAGE 11   **"In dual-earner households, women tend to do twice as much child care and housework as men"**: Bianchi, S. M., Sayer, L. C., Milkie, M. A., & Robinson, J. P. (2012). Housework: Who did, does or will do it, and how much does it matter? *Social Forces, 91*(1), 55–63.

PAGE 11   **"four in ten working mothers report always feeling rushed"**: Who's feeling rushed? (2016, February 28). Pew Research Center. Retrieved from *www.pewsocialtrends.org/2006/02/28/whos-feeling-rushed*.

PAGE 11   **"those who earn more than their male partners actually increase rather than decrease their unpaid labor"**: Bittman, M., England, P., Sayer, L., Folbre, N., & Matheson, G. (2003). When does gender trump money? Bargaining and time in household work. *American Journal of Sociology, 109*(1), 186–214.

PAGE 13   **"please take this test, which is based on the empirically validated Self-Compassion Scale"**: Raes, F., Pommier, E., Neff, K. D., & Van Gucht, D. (2011). Construction and factorial validation of a short form of the Self-Compassion Scale. *Clinical Psychology and Psychotherapy, 18*(3), 250–255.

CHAPTER 2. REPLENISHING OURSELVES: HOW SELF-COMPASSION COMBATS BURNOUT

PAGE 18   **"people who are more self-compassionate benefit in terms of their general mental and physical health"**: Neff, K. D. (2023). Self-compassion: Theory, method, research, and intervention. *Annual Review of Psychology, 74*, 193–218.

PAGE 18   **"using self-report measures like the Self-Compassion Scale and correlating scores with other outcomes"**: Neff, K. D. (2003). The development and validation of a scale to measure self-compassion. *Self and Identity, 2*(3), 223–250.

PAGE 18   **"examining what happens to those who learn to be more self-compassionate by taking a training course like MSC"**: Neff, K. D., & Germer, C. K. (2013). A pilot study and randomized controlled trial of the mindful self-compassion program. *Journal of Clinical Psychology, 69*(1), 28–44.

PAGE 18   **"a lot of research on self-compassion and burnout"**: Rushforth, A., Durk, M., Rothwell-Blake, G. A., Kirkman, A., Ng, F., & Kotera, Y. (2023). Self-compassion interventions to target secondary traumatic stress in healthcare workers: A systematic review. *International Journal of Environmental Research and Public Health, 20*(12), 6109.

See also: Abdollahi, A., Taheri, A., & Allen, K. A. (2021). Perceived stress, self-compassion and job burnout in nurses: the moderating role of self-compassion. *Journal of Research in Nursing, 26*(3), 182–191.

Crego, A., Yela, J. R., Riesco-Matías, P., Gómez-Martínez, M. Á., & Vicente-Arruebarrena, A. (2022). The benefits of self-compassion in mental health professionals: A systematic review of empirical research. *Psychology Research and Behavior Management, 15*, 2599–2620.

Eriksson, T., Germundsjö, L., Åström, E., & Rönnlund, M. (2018). Mindful self-compassion training reduces stress and burnout symptoms among practicing psychologists: A randomized controlled trial of a brief web-based intervention. *Frontiers in Psychology, 9*, 2340.

Liberman, T., Bidegain, M., Berriel, A., López, F. M., Ibarra, A., Pisani, M., . . . & Castelló, M. E. (2024). Effects of a virtual mindful self-compassion training on mindfulness, self-compassion, empathy, well-being, and wtress in Uruguayan primary school teachers during COVID-19 times. *Mindfulness,* 1–15.

Román-Calderón, J. P., Krikorian, A., Ruiz, E., Romero, A. M., & Lemos, M. (2024). Compassion and self-compassion: Counterfactors of burnout in medical students and physicians. *Psychological Reports, 127*(3), 1032–1049.

PAGE 19   **"The Benefits of Self-Compassion"**: Neff, K. D. (2023). Self-compassion: Theory, method, research, and intervention. *Annual Review of Psychology, 74*, 193–218.

PAGE 20   **"research on the efficacy of the brief training"**: Neff, K. D., Knox, M. C., Long, P., & Gregory, K. (2020). Caring for others without losing yourself: An adaptation of the mindful self-compassion program for healthcare communities. *Journal of Clinical Psychology, 76*(9), 1543–1562.

CHAPTER 3. A RECIPE FOR RESILIENCE: THE INGREDIENTS OF SELF-COMPASSION

PAGE 25   **"that work together to help us when we're struggling"**: Neff, K. D. (2003). Self-compassion: An alternative conceptualization of a healthy attitude toward oneself. *Self and Identity, 2*, 85–102.

PAGE 29   **"self-compassion offers strength and resilience"**: Neff, K. D. (2023). Self-compassion: Theory, method, research, and intervention. *Annual Review of Psychology, 74*, 193–218.

PAGE 31   **"the more you practice self-compassion, the more self-compassionate you will become"**: Ferrari, M., Hunt, C., Harrysunker, A., Abbott, M. J., Beath, A. P., &

Einstein, D. A. (2019). Self-compassion interventions and psychosocial outcomes: A meta-analysis of RCTs. *Mindfulness, 10*, 1455–1473.

CHAPTER 4. IT'S NOT WHAT YOU THINK: MISGIVINGS ABOUT SELF-COMPASSION

PAGE 35   **"most of the common worries about self-compassion have been disproven by research":** Most of the research cited in this chapter is summarized in Neff, K. D. (2023). Self-compassion: Theory, method, research, and intervention. *Annual Review of Psychology, 74*, 193–218.

CHAPTER 5. YOUR BODY KNOWS: THE PHYSIOLOGY OF STRESS AND CARE

PAGE 44   **"the damage that chronic stress can do":** McEwen, B. S. (2017). Neurobiological and systemic effects of chronic stress. *Chronic Stress, 1*. Retrieved from *www.ncbi.nlm.nih.gov/pmc/articles/PMC5573220*.

PAGE 46   **"An important way for humans to feel safe is through feelings of warmth and connection":** Porges, S. W. (2022). Polyvagal theory: A science of safety. *Frontiers in Integrative Neuroscience, 16*, 27.

PAGE 46   **"which counteracts sympathetic arousal":** Gilbert, P. (2009). Introducing compassion-focused therapy. *Advances in Psychiatric Treatment, 15*(3), 199–208.

PAGE 47   **"stress-related markers such as inflammation":** Bégin, C., Gilbert-Ouimet, M., & Truchon, M. (2024). Self-compassion, burnout, and biomarkers in a sample of healthcare workers during the COVID-19 pandemic: A cross-sectional correlational study. *Discover Psychology, 4*(1), 75.

PAGE 47   **"self-compassion activates the parasympathetic nervous system":** Slivjak, E. T., Kirk, A., & Arch, J. J. (2023). The psychophysiology of self-compassion. In A. Finlay-Jones, K. Bluth, & K. Neff (Eds.), *Handbook of self-compassion* (pp. 291–307). New York: Springer.

PAGE 47   **"self-compassion is linked to lower perceptions of stress":** Allen, A. B., & Leary, M. R. (2010). Self-compassion, stress, and coping. *Social and Personality Psychology Compass, 4*(2), 107–118.

PAGE 48   **"soothing self-touch such as placing a hand on your own heart":** Kirschner, H., Kuyken, W., Wright, K., Roberts, H., Brejcha, C., & Karl, A. (2019). Soothing your heart and feeling connected: A new experimental paradigm to study the benefits of self-compassion. *Clinical Psychological Science, 7*(3), 545–565.

Dreisoerner, A., Junker, N. M., Schlotz, W., Heimrich, J., Bloemeke, S., Ditzen, B., & van Dick, R. (2021). Self-soothing touch and being hugged reduce cortisol responses to stress: A randomized controlled trial on stress, physical touch, and social identity. *Comprehensive Psychoneuroendocrinology, 8*, 100091.

CHAPTER 8. PUTTING THINGS IN PERSPECTIVE: MINDFUL AWARENESS

PAGE 74 **"the default mode tends to be active when we're not paying attention"**: Raichle, M. E. (2015). The brain's default mode network. *Annual Review of Neuroscience, 38*, 433–447.

PAGE 74 **"the more we practice mindfulness, the less we're trapped in the default mode"**: Brewer, J. A., Worhunsky, P. D., Gray, J. R., Tang, Y. Y., Weber, J., & Kober, H. (2011). Meditation experience is associated with differences in default mode network activity and connectivity. *Proceedings of the National Academy of Sciences, 108*(50), 20254–20259.

PAGE 75 **"the more you practice mindfulness, the more self-compassionate you become"**: Boellinghaus, I., Jones, F. W., & Hutton, J. (2014). The role of mindfulness and loving-kindness meditation in cultivating self-compassion and other-focused concern in health care professionals. *Mindfulness, 5*, 129–138.

CHAPTER 9. RESISTANCE IS FUTILE: HOW FIGHTING BURNOUT MAKES IT WORSE

PAGE 80 **"suppressing unwanted thoughts and feelings just intensifies them"**: Wegner, D. M., Schneider, D. J., Carter, S. R., & White, T. L. (1987). Paradoxical effects of thought suppression. *Journal of Personality and Social Psychology, 53*(1), 5.

PAGE 80 **"Pain × Resistance = Suffering"**: Young, S. (2016). *A pain processing algorithm*. Retrieved from *https://www.shinzen.org/wp-content/uploads/2016/12/art_painprocessingalg.pdf*.

CHAPTER 10. FACING THE STORM: WORKING WITH THE DIFFICULT EMOTIONS OF BURNOUT

PAGE 87 **"when fear is powering our reactions"**: Halifax, J. (2009). *Being with dying: Cultivating compassion and fearlessness in the presence of death*. Boulder, CO: Shambhala Publications.

PAGE 91 **"using this strategy weakens the brain's tendency to become reactive"**: Burklund, L. J., Creswell, J. D., Irwin, M. R., & Lieberman, M. D. (2014). The common and distinct neural bases of affect labeling and reappraisal in healthy adults. *Frontiers in Psychology, 5*, 221.

CHAPTER 11. STOPPING THE DRAIN: REDUCING EMPATHY FATIGUE

PAGE 95 **"a particular type of neuron, called *mirror neurons*"**: Bonini, L., Rotunno, C., Arcuri, E., & Gallese, V. (2022). Mirror neurons 30 years later: Implications and applications. *Trends in Cognitive Sciences, 26*(9), 767–781.

PAGE 95 **"a field sometimes referred to as *interpersonal neurobiology*"**: Schore, A. N.

(2021). The interpersonal neurobiology of intersubjectivity. *Frontiers in Psychology, 12*, 1366.

Hu, Y., Cheng, X., Pan, Y., & Hu, Y. (2022). The intrapersonal and interpersonal consequences of interpersonal synchrony. *Acta Psychologica, 224*(3), 103513.

PAGE 95 **"synchronization occurs between two people":** Kawasaki, M., Yamada, Y., Ushiku, Y., Miyauchi, E., & Yamaguchi, Y. (2013). Inter-brain synchronization during coordination of speech rhythm in human-to-human social interaction. *Scientific Reports, 3*(1), 1692.

PAGE 95 **"the pain centers in our own brains have been activated":** Bernhardt, B. C., & Singer, T. (2012). The neural basis of empathy. *Annual Review of Neuroscience, 35*, 1–23.

PAGE 97 **"The U.S. Department of Health and Human Services describes secondary traumatic stress":** Administration for Children and Families. (2023). Secondary traumatic stress. Retrieved from *www.acf.hhs.gov/trauma-toolkit/secondary-traumatic-stress*.

Bride, B. E., Robinson, M. M., Yegidis, B., & Figley, C. R. (2003). Secondary Traumatic Stress Scale. *Research on Social Work Practice, 14*(1), 27–35.

PAGE 97 **"a research study that trained people in either compassion or empathy":** Singer, T., & Klimecki, O. M. (2014). Empathy and compassion. *Current Biology, 24*(18), R875–R878.

CHAPTER 12. WHEN GOOD ISN'T GOOD ENOUGH: AVOIDING THE PERFECTIONISM SINKHOLE

PAGE 104 **"if you're a perfectionist, you're vulnerable to burnout":** Hill, A. , & Curran, T. (2016). Multidimensional perfectionism and burnout: A meta-analysis. *Personality and Social Psychology Review, 20*(3), 269–288.

PAGE 106 **"perfectionists tend to have what is called *contingent self-esteem*":** Hill, A. P., Hall, H. K., & Appleton, R. (2011). The relationship between multidimensional perfectionism and contingencies of self-worth. *Personality and Individual Differences, 50*(2), 238–242.

PAGE 106 **"our sense of self-worth isn't contingent on success or failure":** Neff, K. D., & Vonk, R. (2009). Self-compassion versus global self-esteem: Two different ways of relating to oneself. *Journal of Personality, 77*(1), 23–50.

PAGE 107 **"self-compassionate people still set high standards for themselves":** Linnett, R. J., & Kibowski, F. (2020). A multidimensional approach to perfectionism and self-compassion. *Self and Identity, 19*(7), 757–783.

PAGE 107 **"a study of how self-compassion training impacted NCAA athletes":** Kuchar, A. L., Neff, K. D., & Mosewich, A. D. (2023). Resilience and Enhancement in Sport, Exercise, & Training (RESET): A brief self-compassion intervention with NCAA student-athletes. *Psychology of Sport and Exercise, 67*, 102426.

PAGE 107 **"Perfectionism is typically a learned behavior stemming from pain in our childhood":** Chen, C., Hewitt, P. L., & Flett, G. L. (2019). Adverse childhood experiences and multidimensional perfectionism in young adults. *Personality and Individual Differences, 146*, 53–57.

CHAPTER 13. WHY WE BEAT OURSELVES UP: UNDERSTANDING THE INNER CRITIC

PAGE 111   **"Self-criticism causes the same physiological changes as any other chronic stressor":** Hering, D., Lachowska, K., & Schlaich, M. (2015). Role of the sympathetic nervous system in stress-mediated cardiovascular disease. *Current Hypertension Reports, 17*, 1–9.

     Albert, P., Rice, K. G., & Caffee, L. (2016). Perfectionism affects blood pressure in response to repeated exposure to stress. *Stress and Health, 32*(2), 157–166.

PAGE 111   **"It's also a major cause of depression":** Dinger, U., Barrett, M. S., Zimmermann, J., Schauenburg, H., Wright, A. G., Renner, F., . . . Barber, J. P. (2015). Interpersonal problems, dependency, and self-criticism in major depressive disorder. *Journal of Clinical Psychology, 71*(1), 93–104.

PAGE 113   **"the biggest block to self-compassion is the belief it will undermine our motivation":** Robinson, K. J., Mayer, S., Allen, A. B., Terry, M., Chilton, A., & Leary, M. R. (2016). Resisting self-compassion: Why are some people opposed to being kind to themselves? *Self and Identity, 15*(5), 505–524.

PAGE 113   **"self-criticism has the same effect":** Werner, A. M., Tibubos, A. N., Rohrmann, S., & Reiss, N. (2019). The clinical trait self-criticism and its relation to psychopathology: A systematic review—update. *Journal of Affective Disorders, 246*, 530–547.

PAGES 114–115   **"children not only internalize the critical messages parents direct at them personally":** Bleys, D., Soenens, B., Boone, L., Claes, S., Vliegen, N., & Luyten, P. (2016). The role of intergenerational similarity and parenting in adolescent self-criticism: An actor–partner interdependence model. *Journal of Adolescence, 49*, 68–76.

PAGE 115   **"a highly effective therapy model called *internal family systems* (IFS)":** Schwartz, R. (2021). *No bad parts.* Louisville, CO: Sounds True.

PAGE 116   **"we can't solve a problem with the same mind that created it":** Rowe, D. E., & Schulmann, R. (Eds.). (2007). *Einstein on politics: His private thoughts and public stands on nationalism, zionism, war, peace, and the bomb.* Princeton, NJ: Princeton University Press.

CHAPTER 14. DOING SOMETHING ABOUT IT: FIERCE SELF-COMPASSION IN ACTION

PAGE 124   **"Power without love is reckless and abusive, and love without power is sentimental and anemic":** King, M. L. K. (1967, August 16). Where do we go from here? Speech delivered at the 11th Convention of the Southern Christian Leadership Conference, Atlanta, Georgia.

PAGE 124 **"Although venting and ruminating on anger is problematic"**: Stapleton, K., Fägersten, K. B., Stephens, R., & Loveday, C. (2022). The power of swearing: What we know and what we don't. *Lingua, 277*, 103406.

CHAPTER 15. DRAWING A LINE IN THE SAND: LEARNING HOW TO SAY NO

PAGE 132 **"self-compassionate people are less likely to subordinate their own needs"**: Yarnell, L. M., & Neff, K. D. (2013). Self-compassion, interpersonal conflict resolutions, and well-being. *Self and Identity, 12*(2), 146–159.

PAGE 135 **"the model of nonviolent communication developed by Marshall Rosenberg is particularly helpful"**: Rosenberg, M. (2015). *Nonviolent communication: A language of life: Life-changing tools for healthy relationships.* Encinitas, CA: PuddleDancer Press.

CHAPTER 16. PROVIDING FOR OURSELVES: WHAT DO I NEED?

PAGES 139–140 **"The Dalai Lama describes compassion as 'wise selfishness'"**: Harris, D. (2023, January 25). The benefits of "wise selfishness." *New York Times.*

PAGES 142–143 **"Winona, who was Navajo, had to struggle with this living in Albuquerque"**: Court rules APS subject to state anti-discrimination laws after teacher called student "a bloody Indian." (2023, June 1). ACLU New Mexico. Retrieved from *www.aclu-nm.org/en/press-releases/court-rules-aps-subject-state-anti-discrimination-laws-after-teacher-called-student.*

PAGE 143 **"most people are more compassionate toward others than themselves"**: Pommier, E., Neff, K. D., & Tóth-Király, I. (2019). The development and validation of the Compassion Scale. *Assessment, 27*(1), 21–39.

PAGE 143 **"women have less self-compassion and more compassion for others than men"**: Yarnell, L. M., Neff, K. D., Davidson, O. A., & Mullarkey, M. (2019). Gender differences in self-compassion: Examining the role of gender role orientation. *Mindfulness, 10*, 1136–1152.

PAGE 143 **"women allow themselves less free time than men and benefit less from it"**: Mattingly, M. J., & Blanchi, S. M. (2003). Gender differences in the quantity and quality of free time: The US experience. *Social Forces, 81*(3), 999–1030.

PAGE 143 **"self-compassionate people are better able to take care of others"**: Lathren, C. R., Rao, S. S., Park, J., & Bluth, K. (2021). Self-compassion and current close interpersonal relationships: A scoping literature review. *Mindfulness, 12*, 1078–1093.

PAGE 143 **"are more adept at compromise, and are more willing to seek a win–win solution"**: Yarnell, L. M., & Neff, K. D. (2013). Self-compassion, interpersonal conflict resolutions, and well-being. *Self and Identity, 12*(2), 146–159.

PAGE 145 **"one of the primary benefits of self-compassion is greater authenticity"**: Zhang, J. W., Chen, S., Tomova Shakur, T. K., Bilgin, B., Chai, W. J., Ramis, T., . . . Manukyan,

A. (2019). A compassionate self is a true self? Self-compassion promotes subjective authenticity. *Personality and Social Psychology Bulletin, 45*(9), 1323–1337.

CHAPTER 17. REDISCOVERING MEANING: WHAT ARE MY CORE VALUES?

PAGE 149   **"the stress of moral injury can contribute to burnout":** Mantri, S., Lawson, J., Wang, Z., & Koenig, H. (2021). Prevalence and predictors of moral injury symptoms in health care professionals. *Journal of Nervous and Mental Disease, 209*(3), 174–180.

PAGE 150   **"we're more likely to criticize and blame ourselves":** Zerach, G., & Levi-Belz, Y. (2022). Moral injury, PTSD, and complex PTSD among Israeli health and social care workers during the COVID-19 pandemic: The moderating role of self-criticism. *Psychological Trauma: Theory, Research, Practice, and Policy, 14*(8), 1314–1323.

PAGE 150   **"self-compassion can help when facing moral injury and softens its impact":** Forkus, S. R., Breines, J. G., & Weiss, N. H. (2019). Morally injurious experiences and mental health: The moderating role of self-compassion. *Psychological Trauma: Theory, Research, Practice, and Policy, 11*(6), 630.

PAGE 150   **"people whose lives are infused with meaning feel more contentment":** Ryff, C. D. (2017). Eudaimonic well-being, inequality, and health: Recent findings and future directions. *International Review of Economics, 64*, 159–178.

PAGE 150   **"living in accord with our values helps us feel authentic":** Smallenbroek, O., Zelenski, J. M., & Whelan, D. C. (2017). Authenticity as a eudaimonic construct: The relationships among authenticity, values, and valence. *Journal of Positive Psychology, 12*(2), 197–209.

PAGE 150   **"core values are central to the acceptance and commitment therapy (ACT) model":** Wilson, K. G., & Murrell, A. R. (2004). Values work in acceptance and commitment therapy: Setting a course for behavioral treatment. In S. C. Hayes, V. M. Follette, & M. M. Linehan (Eds.), *Mindfulness and acceptance: Expanding the cognitive-behavioral tradition* (pp. 120–151). New York: Guilford Press.

PAGE 152   **"If you are always trying to be normal you will never know how amazing you can be":** Maya Angelou, Facebook post, February 5, 2014.

PAGE 154   **"Discovering Your Core Values":** Adapted from the tombstone exercise in acceptance and commitment therapy, as described in Luoma, J. B., Hayes, S. C., & Walser, R. D. (2007). *Learning ACT: An acceptance and commitment therapy skills-training manual for therapists.* Oakland, CA: New Harbinger.

CHAPTER 18. BECOMING A WISE INNER COACH: SELF-COMPASSIONATE MOTIVATION

PAGE 159   **"the study done with NCAA athletes":** Kuchar, A. L., Neff, K. D., & Mosewich, A. D. (2023). Resilience and Enhancement in Sport, Exercise, & Training (RESET): A brief self-compassion intervention with NCAA student-athletes. *Psychology of Sport and Exercise, 67*, 102426.

PAGE 159   **"self-compassionate people tend to have a growth mindset rather than a fixed mindset"**: Kwan, L. Y. Y., Hung, Y. S., & Lam, L. (2022, April). How can we reap learning benefits for individuals with growth and fixed mindsets? Understanding self-reflection and self-compassion as the psychological pathways to maximize positive learning outcomes. *Frontiers in Education, 7,* 800530.

PAGE 159   **"Carol Dweck, a well-known research psychologist who studies learning"**: Dweck, C. S. (2006). *Mindset: The new psychology of success.* New York: Random house.

PAGE 159   **"<u>F</u>riendly, <u>U</u>seful, <u>C</u>alm, <u>K</u>ind"**: Discussion on YouTube. (2020, July 29). Retrieved from *www.youtube.com/watch?v=6g4vkdLXzV4.*

CHAPTER 19. GOODWILL, NOT GOOD FEELINGS: CULTIVATING LOVING-KINDNESS

PAGE 166   **"self-compassionate people tend to be more hopeful and optimistic"**: Neff, K. D., Rude, S. S., & Kirkpatrick, K. L. (2007). An examination of self-compassion in relation to positive psychological functioning and personality traits. *Journal of Research in Personality, 41*(4), 908–916.

PAGE 167   **"practicing traditional loving-kindness meditation increases self-compassion"**: Reilly, E. B., & Stuyvenberg, C. L. (2023). A meta-analysis of loving-kindness meditations on self-compassion. *Mindfulness, 14*(10), 2299–2310.

PAGE 167   **"practicing self-compassion increases joy and happiness"**: Hollis-Walker, L., & Colosimo, K. (2011). Mindfulness, self-compassion, and happiness in non-meditators: A theoretical and empirical examination. *Personality and Individual Differences, 50*(2), 222–227.

PAGE 168   **"Why does Torah tell us to 'place these words upon your hearts'?"**: Palmer, P. J. (2005). *The politics of the brokenhearted: Essays on the deepening of the American dream.* Kalamazoo, MI: Fetzer Institute.

CHAPTER 20. SMALL PLEASURES: SAVORING THE GOOD

PAGE 174   **"our brains are hardwired to pay attention to problems"**: Vaish, A., Grossmann, T., & Woodward, A. (2008). Not all emotions are created equal: The negativity bias in social-emotional development. *Psychological Bulletin, 134*(3), 383.

PAGE 174   **"Velcro for negative information and Teflon for positive information"**: Bergeisen, M. (2010, September 22). The neuroscience of happiness. *Greater Good Magazine.* Retrieved from *https://greatergood.berkeley.edu/article/item/the_neuroscience_of_happiness.*

PAGE 175   **"benefits of positive states of mind like happiness and life satisfaction"**: Seligman, M. E. (2019). Positive psychology: A personal history. *Annual Review of Clinical Psychology, 15,* 1–23.

PAGE 175   **"coined the term *broaden and build*"**: Fredrickson, B. L. (2001). The role of positive emotions in positive psychology: The broaden-and-build theory of positive emotions. *American Psychologist, 56*(3), 218.

PAGE 175 **"one of the benefits of self-compassion is that it counteracts the negativity bias":** Yip, V. T., & Tong, M. W. E. (2021). Self-compassion and attention: Self-compassion facilitates disengagement from negative stimuli. *Journal of Positive Psychology, 16*(5), 593–609.

Neff, K., & Davidson, O. (2016). Self-compassion: Embracing suffering with kindness. In *Mindfulness in positive psychology* (pp. 37–50). Oxfordshire, UK: Routledge.

PAGE 176 **"Compassion itself is a positive emotion":** Förster, K., & Kanske, P. (2022). Upregulating positive affect through compassion: Psychological and physiological evidence. *International Journal of Psychophysiology, 176,* 100–107.

PAGE 176 **"self-compassionate people tend to be more hopeful and optimistic":** Neff, K. D., Rude, S. S., & Kirkpatrick, K. L. (2007). An examination of self-compassion in relation to positive psychological functioning and personality traits. *Journal of Research in Personality, 41*(4), 908–916.

PAGE 176 **"feel more love, joy, gratitude, contentment, hope, pride, interest, amusement, and awe":** Zeng, X., Chiu, C. P., Wang, R., Oei, T. P., & Leung, F. Y. (2015). The effect of loving-kindness meditation on positive emotions: A meta-analytic review. *Frontiers in Psychology, 6,* 1693.

PAGE 177 **"a regular practice of gratitude lifts people up":** Jans-Beken, L., Jacobs, N., Janssens, M., Peeters, S., Reijnders, J., Lechner, L., & Lataster, J. (2020). Gratitude and health: An updated review. *Journal of Positive Psychology, 15*(6), 743–782.

PAGE 177 **"individuals in high-stress jobs who have higher levels of gratitude experience lower levels of burnout":** Lee, J. Y., Kim, S. Y., Bae, K. Y., Kim, J. M., Shin, I. S., Yoon, J. S., & Kim, S. W. (2018). The association of gratitude with perceived stress and burnout among male firefighters in Korea. *Personality and Individual Differences, 123,* 205–208.

PAGE 178 **"Sense and Savor Walk":** Adapted from Bryant, F., & Veroff, J. (2007). *Savoring: A new model of positive experience.* Mahwah, NJ: Erlbaum.

CHAPTER 21. KNOWING OUR STRENGTHS: THE PRACTICE OF SELF-APPRECIATION

PAGE 184 **"A number of character strengths studied in the field of positive psychology":** Peterson, C., & Seligman, M. E. (2004). *Character strengths and virtues: A handbook and classification* (Vol. 1). New York: Oxford University Press.

PAGE 185 **"The deepest principle in human nature is the craving to be appreciated":** James, W. (1981). *The principles of psychology.* Cambridge, MA: Harvard University Press, p. 313. (Original work published 1890)

PAGE 185 **"As Marianne Williamson writes in her book *A Return to Love*":** Williamson, M. (1992). *A return to love: Reflections on the principles of "A course in miracles."* San Francisco: HarperOne, p. 165.

CHAPTER 22. MOVING FORWARD: BECOMING A COMPASSIONATE MESS

PAGE 192   **"to perfect your *love*":** Kornfield, J. (2015, January 14). Freedom of the heart (Episode 11), *Heart wisdom* [podcast]. Retrieved from *https://jackkornfield.com/freedom-heart-heart-wisdom-episode-11*.

PAGE 193   **"the curious paradox is that when I accept myself as I am":** Rogers, C. (1995). *On becoming a person: A therapist's view of psychotherapy*. Boston: Houghton Mifflin, p. 17. (Original work published 1961)

PAGE 193   **"The goal of practice is simply to be a compassionate mess":** Nairn, R. (2009, September). Lecture presented as part of Foundation Training in Compassion. Kagyu Samye Ling Monastery, Dumfriesshire, Scotland.

PAGE 196   **"self-compassion can increase through owning a dog":** Bergen-Cico, D., Smith, Y., Wolford, K., Gooley, C., Hannon, K., Woodruff, R., . . . Gump, B. (2018). Dog ownership and training reduces post-traumatic stress symptoms and increases self-compassion among veterans: Results of a longitudinal control study. *Journal of Alternative and Complementary Medicine, 24*(12), 1166–1175.

PAGE 196   **"doing yoga":** Crews, D. A., Stolz-Newton, M., & Grant, N. S. (2016). The use of yoga to build self-compassion as a healing method for survivors of sexual violence. *Journal of Religion and Spirituality in Social Work: Social Thought, 35*(3), 139–156.

PAGE 196   **"immersing yourself in nature":** Swami, V., Barron, D., Hari, R., Grover, S., Smith, L., & Furnham, A. (2019). The nature of positive body image: Examining associations between nature exposure, self-compassion, functionality appreciation, and body appreciation. *Ecopsychology, 11*(4), 243–253.

PAGE 196   **"going to therapy":** Germer, C. (2023). Self-compassion in psychotherapy: Clinical integration, evidence base, and mechanisms of change. In A. Finlay-Jones, K. Bluth, & K. Neff (Eds.), *Handbook of self-compassion* (pp. 379–415). New York: Springer.

PAGE 196   **"learning mindfulness":** Keng, S. L., Smoski, M. J., Robins, C. J., Ekblad, A. G., & Brantley, J. G. (2012). Mechanisms of change in mindfulness-based stress reduction: Self-compassion and mindfulness as mediators of intervention outcomes. *Journal of Cognitive Psychotherapy, 26*(3), 270–280.

PAGE 196   **"giving support to others":** Breines, J. G., & Chen, S. (2013). Activating the inner caregiver: The role of support-giving schemas in increasing state self-compassion. *Journal of Experimental Social Psychology, 49*(1), 58–64.

PAGE 196   **"taking a long walk":** Steininger, Y., Braun, A., & Morgenroth, O. (2023). Becoming self-compassionate step by step—a field study on the effect of long-distance walking on self-compassion in hikers traveling the Camino Francés. *Mindfulness, 14*(1), 101–112.

PAGE 196   **"Just about anything we do for ourselves":** Susman, E. S., Chen, S., Kring, A. M., & Harvey, A. G. (2024). Daily micropractice can augment single-session interventions: A randomized controlled trial of self-compassionate touch and examining their associations with habit formation in US college students. Behaviour Research and Therapy, 104498.

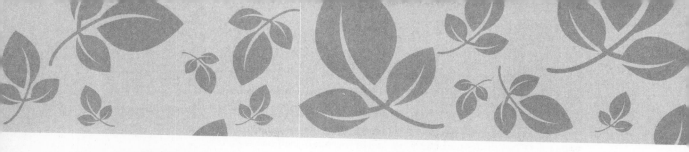

INDEX

ABOUT THE AUTHORS

Kristin Neff, PhD, is Associate Professor of Educational Psychology at The University of Texas at Austin and a pioneer in the field of self-compassion research. She has been recognized as one of the most influential researchers in psychology worldwide. Her books with Christopher Germer include *The Mindful Self-Compassion Workbook: A Proven Way to Accept Yourself, Build Inner Strength, and Thrive* (for the general public) and *Teaching the Mindful Self-Compassion Program: A Guide for Professionals.* Along with Christopher Germer, Dr. Neff developed the empirically supported Mindful Self-Compassion program and founded the Center for Mindful Self-Compassion. Her website is *https://self-compassion.org.*

Christopher Germer, PhD, is a clinical psychologist and Lecturer on Psychiatry (part-time) at Harvard Medical School. His books with Kristin Neff include *The Mindful Self-Compassion Workbook* and *Teaching the Mindful Self-Compassion Program.* Dr. Germer is also author of *The Mindful Path to Self-Compassion* and coeditor of *Mindfulness and Psychotherapy* and *Wisdom and Compassion in Psychotherapy.* He lectures and leads workshops internationally and has a small psychotherapy practice in Massachusetts. His website is *https://chrisgermer.com.*